Research Partners with Lived Experience

Andrew Stranieri • Grant Meredith
Selena Firmin

Editors

Research Partners with Lived Experience

Stories from Patients and Survivors

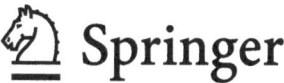 Springer

Editors
Andrew Stranieri
Institute of Innovation, Science
and Sustainability
Federation University
Ballarat, VIC, Australia

Grant Meredith
Global Professional School
Federation University
Ballarat, VIC, Australia

Selena Firmin
Institute of Innovation, Science
and Sustainability
Federation University
Ballarat, VIC, Australia

ISBN 978-981-97-0035-6   ISBN 978-981-97-0033-2   (eBook)
https://doi.org/10.1007/978-981-97-0033-2

This Springer imprint is published by the registered company Springer Nature Singapore Pte Ltd.
The registered company address is: 152 Beach Road, #21-01/04 Gateway East, Singapore 189721,
Singapore

Paper in this product is recyclable.

Foreword

This innovative and fascinating book, *Research Partners with Lived Experience: Stories from Patients and Survivors*, comprises personal narratives of researchers about how experiencing a little-understood condition led them to explore it further with research. "Lived experience," then, refers to first-hand understanding of a condition or problem, in contrast to knowledge obtained from other sources. The conditions experienced by the narrators are wide ranging, relating predominantly to health/allied health, and the progress reportedly made by them through research is inspirational. Importantly, the narratives send the clear message that teams conducting research into human conditions will benefit from having members who can contribute personal insights, as garnered through lived experience.

Australian Stuttering Research Centre   Ann Packman
University of Technology Sydney
Ultimo, NSW, Australia

Preface

Compiling this book has been a journey of awakening for the editors. We were initially motivated to collate experiences of researchers whose personal, intense experiences have led to their research efforts, after reflecting on our own journeys. Articles published on this growing trend tend to focus on patients with lived experience in clinical research teams to illustrate the benefits for individuals and research groups; however, the journey from patient to researcher seems rarely to be intentional or smooth. Soon after the call for expressions of interest for chapters, it became clear that there were experiences beyond the patient narrative alone.

We wanted particularly to gather narratives of diverse journeys so that readers at various stages in their own journey, and established researchers interacting with colleagues with lived experiences, could both glean a deep sense of our authors' lived experiences, empathize, and more completely understand how the experiences triggered quests into research.

We did not anticipate the deeply moving accounts that arrived on our desks. Nor did we anticipate how the act of drafting a submission transformed some authors, including ourselves, in ways that caught them by surprise.

The chapters in this book are not primarily intended to provide an academic treatise about the lived-experience phenomenon. Rather, the chapters reveal personal stories of the transitions authors made from their intense experiences to research endeavours. We hope that the reader can appreciate how each story is unique and collectively illustrates that transitions cannot be readily generalized with cookie-cutter templates. For example, Grant Meredith's stuttering was not linked to his self-identity until later in life when, as an academic, he naturally gravitated to research that supported people who stutter. In contrast, Sherin Tresa Paul's asthma from childhood dramatically shaped every aspect of her life.

For some contributors, the lived experience was as a caregiver. Frada Burstein shifted her research focus from decision science to health informatics following experiences with health care information systems as a caregiver for her elderly father. Jet van der Voet gives us a particularly moving insight into the impact her son's leukaemia had on her. For some authors, the intense lived experience did not involve medical care. Elisa Zentveld and Leo Brunelle share insights into family violence from quite different lived experiences.

Truus Teunissen masterfully interweaves two stories: juxtaposing his reality of life with multiple chronic conditions with aspirations towards scientific endeavour motivated by a deep sense of justice. Leading Dutch researcher, Tineke Abma, shows her tremendous support for patients with lived experience, including Truus and Jet, transitioning to make impacts on research teams.

Marie-Claire Seely's account of debilitating Postural Orthostatic Tachycardia Syndrome led to her return to undergraduate study and ultimately to laboratory-based research. Karen Raymond shows us how Zebras with Spots can commence university studies in their mid-forties and launch future research endeavours off a perfect grade point average. The path from patient to researcher took a different tack for Armita Zarnegar, who had already completed doctoral research in bioinformatics to refocus on digital health.

What is the reader to reap from the chapters? A compelling trend that emerges from the chapters, for us as editors, is a deep appreciation of the capacity of individuals to respond positively when confronted with great adversity. We have found the narratives inspirational and feel a sense of privilege that the authors have shared their journey.

Perhaps the most important concept that a reader may take from the submissions is an invitation to reflect on their own journeys and a deeper appreciation of the importance of acknowledging our own lived experience in our research efforts.

Andrew, Grant and Sally (Editors)

Ballarat, VIC, Australia	Andrew Stranieri
Ballarat, VIC, Australia	Sally Firmin
Ballarat, VIC, Australia	Grant Meredith

Contents

Paradigm Shift: The Lived Experience of a Researcher with Postural Orthostatic Tachycardia Syndrome

Marie-Claire Seeley

Abstract Postural orthostatic tachycardia syndrome (POTS) is a poorly recognised but frequently experienced autonomic nervous system dysfunction. Females of child-bearing age are disproportionately affected, and the syndrome is associated with high disability. POTS has an elusive aitiology but is increasingly recognised as having an immune association and is often triggered by varying environmental factors including viral infection and trauma. This chapter will focus on the narrative story of the diagnostic and research odyssey of the author. Using Kolb's experiential learning cycle, this narrative will reflect on concrete examples of experience to abstract conceptualisations of improved research practices that value and esteem the lived experience of peer researchers with chronic illness (Kolb D. Experiential learning: experience as the source of learning and development. Upper Saddle River: Prentice Hall; 1984). The chapter will detail lessons learned about the historical limitations of the medical model and, in particular, the reasons behind the failings of the traditional positivist approach to research. It will detail the challenges of entrenched gender stereotypes and societal attitudes towards chronic health while following the author's transition from patient to health professional to researcher. Finally, the narrative will articulate the benefits and limitations of 'lived experience' and why it is integral to the progressive research methodology.

Keywords Postural orthostatic tachycardia syndrome · Chronic illness · Research models · Lived experience · Patient researcher · Positivist paradigm · Biomedical model

M.-C. Seeley (✉)
Australian Dysautonomia and Arrhythmia Research Collaboration, The University of Adelaide, Adelaide, SA, Australia
e-mail: marie-claire.seeley@adelaide.edu.au

© The Author(s), under exclusive license to Springer Nature Singapore Pte Ltd. 2024
A. Stranieri et al. (eds.), *Research Partners with Lived Experience*,
https://doi.org/10.1007/978-981-97-0033-2_1

1 The Experience of Chronic Illness

1.1 The First Revelation

It was December 1993 and mid-winter in Central Asia, where my husband Jon and I had been living for the past six months, when we embarked on a gruelling journey by bus from our home in Tashkent, Uzbekistan, to Alma Ata (Almaty) in Kazakhstan, some 800 km to the east. We had heard through our network that an Australian doctor was visiting the region and was willing to see foreign nationals. Central Asia had not long been liberated from the Soviet Union, complicating the already uncomfortable journey with bureaucratic and physical obstacles.

We arrived late in the evening and had to trudge through freshly fallen snow to the entry of one of the dozens of Soviet-style high-rise concrete apartment buildings on the city's outskirts. We stayed with a young Australian couple we knew through mutual friends. A pounding heart, tight chest, and the oppressive feeling of 'air hunger' accompanied every step I took. These symptoms had dogged me for the previous 9 months and were why we had come.

I hadn't always felt this way. Before February 1993, when my symptoms started, I considered myself something of an athlete. I enjoyed good health and had excelled at several sports as a child and teenager, representing my school, region, and occasionally my state. My penchant for independence and adventure in my early twenties led me to Europe and eventually to work in the Eastern Block when revolution swept the communist states behind the iron curtain. With youthful confidence, I was initially oblivious to the risks inherent in travelling there. Intimidating border delays, robberies, and threats of violence increased my vigilance, but still, I was largely unencumbered by what might be called 'normal' fear and anxiety. On reflection, my younger self was somewhat unperturbable in nature.

Yet here I was only months later in this foreign city in the makeshift office of an Australian General Practitioner (GP), experiencing symptoms that felt physically like anxiety but without any apparent emotional instigator for the symptoms. A short walk across a park in the snow on a cold winter's night had made my legs feel like lead while my lungs screamed for air. In retrospect, we rather naively believed that what we thought to be an obvious symptom of a heart problem would be equally apparent to a doctor. I was certain that the problem would be identified, a diagnosis made and a solution to my health problems forthcoming. After all, the only barrier to diagnosis and treatment was the lack of access to a medical professional. The barrier removed; the problem solved. Or so I thought.

After some pleasantries, I detailed the events of the last months. Following a 24-hour stopover in a tropical city in Asia, Jon had first woken with a temperature and a stiff neck. He developed a high fever over the ensuing hours, and I was soon to follow with an equally high temperature and a strange stiffness in my jaw. There were no other symptoms, and being determined and young, we continued our daily tasks, only slightly thwarted by the inconvenience of tiredness, muscle aches, and nightly fevers. A few days later, we were sitting in the front row of an event. I had been feeling the occasional dizziness often associated with illness, but as I sat still, this feeling grew. My vision blurred, and I felt and heard a sudden roaring of static in my ears. I could feel a hot flush running from my chest and up to my face, and I knew with certainty that I was about to faint or vomit. I escaped to the foyer, blinded by black spots in my vision as I walked. Jon soon sat down by my side as I tried to explain what had happened. Once seated, my vision returned, but the breathlessness and thumping headache remained. I stood again after some minutes, thinking the worst was over. It wasn't. Every time I stood, I heard the same deafening roar, my vision faded, and my lungs struggled for air. This experience became my intermittent yet steadfast companion for the following months and years. It took me some time to realise the experiences were purely posture related. I had no medical training and could barely take my pulse. Nevertheless, I soon realised that the sensations were accompanied by a racing heart, which calmed as soon as I sat or lay down. I was vigilant in checking my pulse and frequently found it was too fast to count. When I could discriminate the rate, I would write it down and ask my more medically minded friends whether it was 'normal' to have a heart rate of 180 beats/min when standing still. The answer was always a resounding no!

So now here we were in Central Asia, sitting in front of an experienced doctor in whom I'd placed great hope. I remember his manner was distant. He showed no surprise as we detailed the story of the virus, the fevers, and the ongoing high heart rates and their association with intractable fatigue, shortness of breath, and an inability to do almost anything without extreme exhaustion. He wrote silently, head down, occasionally looking up to ask a question. He gave nothing away in his expression or tone of voice, and I can recall my increasing uneasiness. It was clear my case was not being heard. The judge I sat before had already determined my fate, and nothing I said or did would change his mind. As I had nothing to lose at that point, I got to my feet and asked him if he would take my pulse and blood pressure again. I stood awkwardly, vision lost, heart pounding, lungs screaming, waiting for his response. There was none. He barely glanced at me and mumbled something unintelligible. His tone of voice told me he was having none of it. I can't even remember how the consult ended, except that I left with an overwhelming sense of disappointment and hopelessness. We weren't given any direction, solution or even a comment of 'I'm sorry, I don't know what is wrong with you'. It was clear some judgement had been made, but it remained unspoken, rendered of insufficient importance to convey to me the patient. We were dismissed.

The next morning, we gathered in the kitchen with our hosts discussing our return to Tashkent. One of them, a young female doctor, asked us how the consult went. It was difficult to respond, but I gave a vague reply with no real answer to what was happening. She paused, sheepishly asking, "do you suffer from anxiety?" Jon laughed out loud behind me. I responded, still a little confused by the question. 'No, not at all!' She seemed relieved and continued. 'No, I didn't think that was it either'. And then it dawned on me that that was the unexpressed judgement the doctor had made. He **thought this was anxiety,** and he told our host so, but he hadn't had the courage to say those words to me, even when I stood before him, seeking his opinion and expertise. Instead, he discussed it behind closed doors with another doctor who was not involved in my care. This was a practice I later came to realise is as common as it is inappropriate.

On reflection, I recognised his uneasiness. In his mind, 'anxiety' was akin to shame. It was something he was embarrassed to convey to me, the patient. It was better for him to evade the issue and hope he never saw me again. I was confused. Where in our brief interaction did he have time to assess me for anxiety? There was no questioning of my usual state of mind, no exploring of thought processes or traumas that might indicate environmental triggers for such a strong and sudden onset of physical symptoms. How could he then be so resolute in determining the cause of my suffering? The more I replayed the consult in my mind, the more I realised his judgement was not determined through my interaction; it was made long before I walked in the door. It was independent of me and constructed from his preconceived biases and beliefs about what I represented. He had not consulted with me, the patient, but rather reached back into the schema of his mind where he stored memories of 'people like me' and found his answer. I was a young female suffering from fatigue and weight loss symptoms. To him, the diagnosis needed no critical examination. It could only be one thing.

1.2   The Second Revelation

Some months later, we returned to Australia for answers to my medical conundrum, only to find that every consultation echoed our previous experience. Each doctor sat on the other side of the desk, telling us that, in all likelihood, my affliction was 'in my head'. They shared the same reluctance to utter the word 'anxiety', and each appeared to cast a sympathetic nod towards Jon as he tried to counter their claims. None appeared to show any interest or sympathy for my plight. Nor did they take up the offer to measure my pulse lying and standing. Finally, through persistence, we secured testing with a cardiologist, and I undertook two days of ambulatory heart monitoring.

The weather was hot in Adelaide, and although I hadn't made the connection, my symptoms peaked due to the heat. When we returned to the specialist's office to discuss the results, we discovered that, unlike the others, he was not so encumbered by embarrassment. Rather he detailed his theory in stunning frankness. Firstly, he discussed the monitor results. They appeared to show my heart rate was a normal 50–60 beats per minute (bpm) while resting and sleeping, but it then escalated to a range of between 150 and 200 bpm during my symptomatic periods. I experienced a moment of relief, thinking that, finally, we had the evidence needed to prove my 'innocence'; this wasn't a psychogenic condition but rather a physiological driver caused by postural change. What appeared as an observable, objective marker to us seemed to be of no consequence to him. 'There is nothing wrong with you. You're just a bit anxious', came his summation. 'If this is anxiety, why does it dissipate as soon as I lie down? Surely if I'm anxious, I'll be anxious no matter my position?' I asked. Unfazed by this logic, he continued with his former line of discussion and then, as if to add weight to his 'diagnosis', he said, '**we are taught about young women like you in medical school**'. And there was the second revelation. The creator of the shared schema was not repeated experience and studied expertise; rather, it resulted from an entrenched belief passed from one generation of clinicians to another. What exactly was it that they were 'taught' about *me*? After all, I didn't appear in any textbook. I hadn't been examined or questioned by any professor. How was it that each doctor I met was certain they knew my story and experience?

I resolved never to speak to another doctor about my 'illness'. It seemed futile to continue seeking assistance from a medical system with no logical answers or interest in seeking them. In any case, it was clear that whatever was afflicting me wasn't intent on or capable of killing me, at least not in the short term. Rather it was trying to crush me from within, thwarting my ability to engage in everyday activities and leaving me exhausted after the simplest of tasks. Its arrival plagued my body with only what *I* could feel and experience, leaving no trace for the outside world to observe except for my apparent reluctance to engage in physical activities. It was, in every aspect, an invisible illness.

1.3   The Turning Point

> As long as stress and psychological strain are feminine coded, and a hierarchy between somatic and psychological findings exists in health care, there is a risk that not only the dichotomy between men's and women's pain but also between somatic and psychological conditions are further consolidated (Samulowitz et al. 2018, p. 5).

If there's one thing that children bring, it's the certainty of frequent interactions with illness and doctors. In a long line of negative experiences with clinicians, several were defining moments for my future direction as a nurse and researcher.

Perhaps the most memorable was the day I sat with my screaming, writhing 15-month-old while an elderly locum doctor explained that my child's behaviour was more a reflection of my emotional state than my child's physical health. I was never quite sure where these suppositions came from. I rarely showed much emotion during consults and was prone to internalising my thoughts. Nevertheless, the projections of hysteria persisted.

It was the late 1990s, and we were living in the UK. Our daughter had barely slept a full night since her birth. Her weight fluctuated with every long bout of diarrhoea. The diarrhoea was accompanied by what we could only assume by her writhing and screaming was severe abdominal pain. Repeated doctor visits only elicited comments to the effect that 'anxious mothers create anxious babies'. Finally, I turned to the Internet, which was relatively new at the time and proved revelatory. My daughter's symptoms were clear: pale, foul-smelling diarrhoea with abdominal distension and pain. I was certain it was coeliac disease. Later sitting in the doctor's surgery, steadfast in my conviction and armed with this new information, above the din of my screaming daughter I persisted with requesting a referral for a blood test. The doctor audibly sighed as he opened a drawer, withdrew a pad and started scribbling. As he handed me the referral, he said something that summed up his prejudice and my experience with doctors to date; "**Just so you know, I'm treating your paranoia, not your child's illness!**"

Several weeks later, we were called to the local children's hospital where a paediatrician reluctantly agreed to the blood test while insisting it was highly unlikely that our daughter had coeliac disease, as it was 'very rare'. It took another couple of months before we received a call to return and discuss the results. We were told that the antibodies on our daughter's blood test were 'through the roof'. She was diagnosed with coeliac disease and placed on a lifelong gluten-free diet. No mention or acknowledgement was made of previous discussions by either the paediatrician or the GP. Nevertheless, the experience awakened something in me. I had a new understanding of my power as a consumer of health. I could assess, identity, research, and test hypotheses. The result was both rewarding and validating. It was the beginning of my new journey.

1.4   The Road to Discovery

Not long after this incident, I returned to education and studied health. The Internet had opened up a new world, while experiences with my own and my children's health had revealed both my ability and proclivity for critical enquiry. I had no lofty ambitions, just a drive to understand and find solutions to the problems with which I had been faced. There wasn't an expectation that I could cure myself or change the entire health system, but I felt I might be able to counter the prejudices and maltreatment I had experienced as a health consumer. After a move back to Australia and at the mature age of 33, I entered university to study a Bachelor of Science in Nursing. The next 4 years were a whirlwind of study, juggling kids, placements, and a move interstate. While my own health could still be unpredictable, I was far more adept at managing it.

I continued to scour the Internet for any clues to the cause of my debilitating array of symptoms, until I came across a little-known condition that reflected my experiences to a T. So, it finally had a name, and that name was not 'anxiety', it was postural orthostatic tachycardia syndrome or POTS. I experienced an overwhelming sense of relief; I had been dismissed and disparaged for years, and the proof of my veracity was now sitting right in front of me. It was more than an answer to my health crisis. It was validation of my lived experience and that of so many others. Even so, I felt strangely reticent to search further, as though I might compound the hurt and disappointment caused by years of conflict with the system I was now working in. For the moment, knowing the name would suffice.

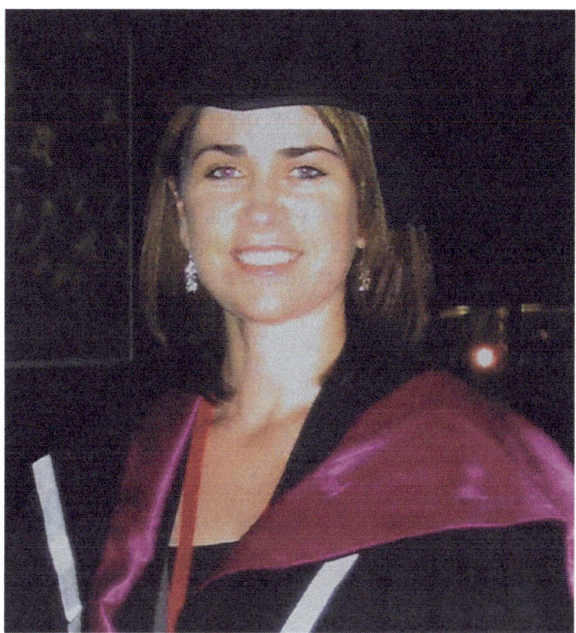

Bachelor of nursing graduation ceremony 2006

Despite this reservation, I set up an automatic alert on a database search and continued to monitor the articles with interest. With each new study came some added understanding of my situation. My fluctuations in weight, fatigue, brain fog, persistently dry eyes, and fluctuating vision were all associated with this syndrome. The problem stemmed from the autonomic nervous system, which is key to managing all the body's unconscious functions, including gut motility, sweat function, blood pressure, and heart rate response (Wells et al. 2017). Disappointingly, no one seemed to know the cause of the condition. Still, a careful review of the available literature revealed the occurrence of a premorbid viral infection to be a common observation and a likely trigger. I kept the articles in a file, which I opened occasionally and continued with my work and life, content for the time being to have it confirmed that I was not malingering.

1.5 The Positivist Ideology

By this time in my career, I had succumbed to the ideology and orthodoxy of the biomedical model. I believed the mantra that patients should generally be seen as passive research participants; their own experiences would prejudice and obscure the 'true' scientific facts of the case, resulting in 'unreliable' findings. I reflected on my situation and concluded that it would be 'irresponsible' to be involved in researching the condition I had personally experienced. After all, every concept explored and variable investigated would be tainted with my own experience and would be seen through the lens of my own pain and illness. Somehow, I believed the positivist dogma that my intimate experience of this illness would hide the 'truth' of its cause. As if the 'truth' was one single entity, a solitary, organic creature that was willfully hiding from view, detectable only to those without the stain of experience to blind their eyes to its existence. My conversion to the theory was as gradual and occult as it was unexamined and unchallenged. On reflection, I can't understand what it was that I thought my experience might obscure. Nevertheless, I kept my distance and turned my mind towards other research that was more removed from my daily experiences.

1.6 The Kind Words

When the medical encounter consists of curiosity, empathy, validation, and a willingness to problem solve, there are fewer distressed patients. (Dr. Ingela Thune-Boyle)

Much happened between 2006 and 2018 to shape my transition to a POTS researcher. Not least of these was the sudden and dramatic onset of gastric dysmotility and fainting in my eldest daughter after she had a short-lived viral illness at the age of 14. It was clearly POTS, and this time there was no choice but to persist and get some help. Initially, we were greeted with the usual dismissive comments about age, gender, and the likelihood it was anxiety related. However, it was clear to me that there was a viral precipitant to her illness. I was sure her condition was physiological and that it demanded a medical response.

Sitting at my desk at Monash University (where I was now working as a nursing academic), I was confused about some of my daughter's other symptoms, which I had not previously associated with POTS. She had multiple dislocations of her joints since she was a toddler and had experienced ongoing joint pain dismissed as 'growing pains' but which still persisted. At the age of 13 she had required her coccyx to be removed due to excessive pain. The surgeon explained to us after the surgery, with some mixture of excitement and confusion, that the coccyx was 'abnormally hypermobile'. I undertook a broader database search using the terms 'hypermobility' and 'postural tachycardia'. Ehlers Danlos Syndrome came up on my screen, and the last piece of the puzzle was revealed.

Ehlers-Danlos Syndrome (EDS) describes a broad range of heritable collagen disorders. Among them is a 'benign' hypermobile type which is accompanied by a plethora of symptoms that plagued our family, including multiple non-traumatic joint dislocations, abnormal scarring, anatomical valvular laxities (including ureteric reflux and mitral valve prolapses), scoliosis, disproportional height to arm span ratio, multiple re-occurring hernias, and a tendency to bleeding (Malfait et al. 2017). By the end of the day, I had a name of a specialist and wrote to him outlining my daughter's problems. He responded quickly, and a month later my daughter and I sat in front of him awaiting the results of the many investigations. He confirmed that she had POTS and EDS and apparently so did I. For good measure he threw in the words **'it's real and it's not in your head'**.

1.7   The Challenge of the Impossible

power (is) not only... a productive force which shapes discourse but also... a presence obscuring certain subjectivities and silencing the voices of those in the relevant positions. (Gillett 2004)

Diagnosis of chronic illness does not equate with curative treatment. Accompanying the relief of validation is invariably the grief associated with acceptance of an uncertain future living with chronic illness. Despite the claims of the doctor from so many years before "learning about women like me" the truth was that Australian medical schools had neglected to include autonomic deregulatory disorders in their curriculum. Instead, the "learning" these doctors referred to was more the type that was whispered in hospital hallways and mentioned or implied discretely in ward meetings and patient handovers. Having worked for some years in Emergency Departments I had been privy to these conversations and innuendos. Patients frequently presented concerned about their racing heart, fatigue, and crumbling functionality. Amongst clinicians' euphemisms such as 'psychosomatic condition', 'functional disorder', 'conversion syndrome', and 'contested illness' were used. Patients were turned away with little in the way of answers and often with a discharge letter pointing to 'non-organic' causes of their symptoms. The evidence for such assertions seemed entirely inconsistent with what I could interpret in the emerging medical literature on POTS. Here I found evidence of organic origins. Dysregulation of the renin-angiotensin aldosterone system, vascular insufficiency with poor cardiac preload, and evidence of altered cerebral perfusion were all documented in the literature. This evidence and my own experience confirmed in my own mind that the condition was very much organic in nature. And yet the knowledge gap and desire for understanding appeared absent in the clinical setting. I saw little hope of a systemic change in attitude and felt powerless to do anything except reassure those seeking help that it wasn't 'in their head'. Largely, I kept a low profile believing the problem was insurmountable and that I had no real capacity to bring about change as an individual. Much to my shame, even though I had decided to pursue a master's in research as part of my academic nursing role, I deliberately chose to steer away from exploring the condition I knew best.

1.8   The Final Revelation

The history of science is a tale of multifarious shifting of allegiance from theory to theory. (Smith 1986)

In 2018 I continued to dabble in academic work and found myself teaching varying undergraduate research methodology courses. Our family had recently moved interstate, and I continued to hang on to the hope that I might stumble across the right supervisor to help me engage in POTS research. Coincidentally, at this time, I was probably the healthiest I had been since I was a young athletic teenager. Having taken up trail running, I had lost some weight and was revelling in return to my youthful fitness. A few months out from my 50th birthday, I was running in the hills and stopped at the crest of a hill to survey the view and contemplate my healthy transformation. Maybe this was what I needed all along, a return to some hard-hitting exercise. The euphoria however was short-lived. Two days later I returned to the same trail run only this time I was revisited by the pounding heart and characteristic air hunger of old. My smart watch began flashing warnings of tachycardia and I felt a heavy pressure in my central chest. I stopped, rested, and returned to the car defeated.

It was a rapid slide to incapacity. Within days I was struggling to make it to the bathroom with any semblance of normal vision. When I got there I would sit on the floor of the shower, the only safe place if I was to avoid a faint. Simple tasks became difficult as I struggled to stand or sit upright. This time the doctors were far more responsive and concerned. None questioned my motives or my sex and all worked with some level of sympathy and respect to try to find a cause for my sudden deterioration. It was a refreshing and comforting change. I wondered if the attitude had anything to do with my developed ability to command a language they understood. Rather than speaking in vagaries about my 'thumping heart' and my 'roaring ears' I was able to articulate the appropriate medical terminology. Instead, I talked of tachycardia, hyperadrenergic responses, and the unusual and sudden onset of polyuria, which had beset me.

Within a matter of weeks, I had lost several kilos as well as my capacity to think clearly. One day, in an effort to remain functional, I took a slow walk around the block from my house. This was a route I was very familiar with but soon, I was lost, unable to find the way home even with the help of my phone and google maps. I sat on the kerb and did the only thing I had capacity for; I cried.

Months of hospitalisations and treatments ensued before I was able to recover any significant level of functioning. During this process, I had many hours to contemplate my silent assailant. When I could think, I would pore over recent journal articles looking for therapies that might help. It took courage, but I managed to raise some of these treatment options with my doctors, and through trial and error, they got me on therapies that helped me recover. This experience induced the realisation that being both patient and researcher was not a hindrance to an empirical scientific investigation but an advantage I needed to exploit.

POTS, like so many chronic illnesses, is hard to measure objectively. Elevated heart rate is one simple but inadequate quantification behind a veritable feast of nervous system regulatory dysfunctions. I became mindful that it took great faith from my physicians to believe what invariably they couldn't see. Nausea, dizziness, brain fog, and fatigue were all immeasurable symptoms of my suffering. I was essentially a fit and healthy middle-aged woman by all other objective measures.

How, then, could a solution be found for POTS if the symptoms of the condition were not extractable, measurable, and able to be scientifically explored? The inadequacy of the biomedical model to address the syndrome I suffered was laid bare. The truth was that "...when the disease agent perspective is transferred from infectious to chronic diseases, the weaknesses of the (biomedical) model is even more sharply apparent" (Dean 2004).

My gradual recovery coincided with the global descent into chaos as the SARS-CoV-2 pandemic swept the globe, creating a paradox from which several revelations emerged. First, an earnest desire to return to clinical nursing beset me, followed by what seemed an urgent need to pay attention to what I deemed to be an inevitable tsunami of post-viral autonomic disorders coming our way. In the midst of all of this, I discovered the most curious of things. Despite the widespread illness and the global medical crisis, the pandemic had thrown me a lifeline. Chronic ill-health felt akin to following others on a trail run who are fitter and faster than yourself; You were always alone and behind the pack. You could see them; if they thought to look behind, they would also see you. However, most of the time was spent on your own, hoping to make it to the next bend. But now, in the middle of a pandemic, it was as if the whole pack had stopped for a rest, and I could finally join them. There were no places to be, no exhaustion to hide. Just plenty of time to share and think and have companionship again. The hidden blessing of the pandemic was that it allowed me to dare hope that I might have a contribution to make again to society. That there was still time to be of benefit.

It was about this time I came across a cardiologist interested in POTS. I had seen his name some years before in an article and, as he lived in the same city, had thought of contacting him to discuss his work. As fate would have it, we met through another forum. He recognised my insight into the syndrome and challenged me to use my clinical and research background to study further. It took me some months to consider the proposition. There were many reasons not to do it, mostly related to my age and illness. But upon thorough examination, none of them held any weight. What did I have to lose? The greatest barrier remained my unpredictable health. This I declared upfront, knowing full well that even those with the keenest interest and knowledge about POTS, could not quite grasp the difficulty of maintaining some semblance of reliability when living with chronic illness. Nevertheless, I strode forward, eyes open, into research.

2   The Reflections of a Pilgrim

2.1   Finding a Voice

A common dilemma in gender research involves how to create awareness about stereotypes without confirming or reinforcing them. (Samulowitz et al. 2018)

Within months I was enrolled in a PhD programme at the University of Adelaide. My topic: 'autonomic dysfunction in post-acute sequelae of COVID-19'. Astoundingly, within 3 months of starting, I had secured some funding, completed the necessary ethics requirements and was ready to enroll my first participant. As predicted, the dysautonomia wave crashed upon our shores. By the end of 2022, multiple studies reported a rise in POTS presentations following COVID-19 infection. As a result, my first 2 years of research were a whirlwind of productivity that forced, by necessity, a rapid transition from patient to researcher.

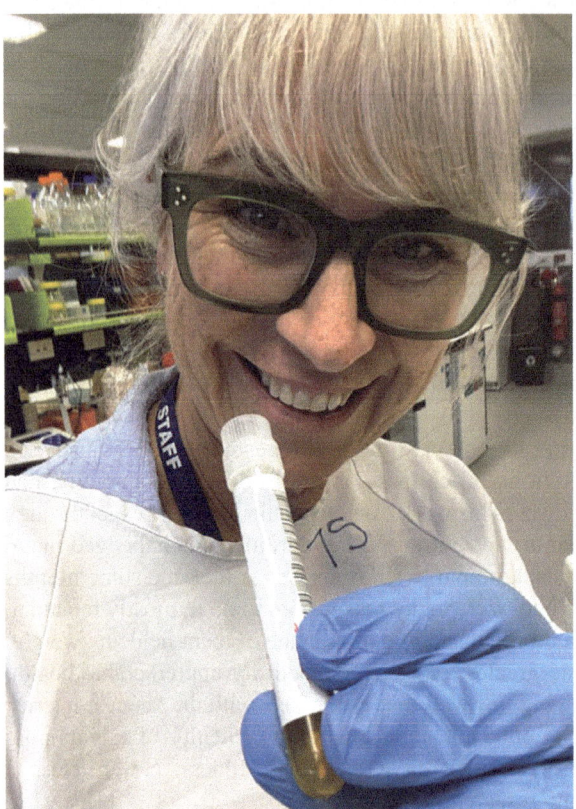

December 2022, preparing serum samples for storage

The patient/researcher has many unique hurdles and challenges to contend with. Not least is the tendency to assume others will discount your opinions because of your experience. It is easy for distrust to creep in as a response to previous medical experiences. This drove much of my interaction with doctors in the preceding decades. I assumed the worst motives and interpreted every question in the light of the previous prejudices displayed. This tendency occasionally compromised my health as I felt I would rather stay silent and die quietly than give another doctor the satisfaction of saying I was 'just anxious'. I also learned to play the game, as I saw it, by not revealing too many symptoms to any doctor lest they perceive me as 'attention seeking'. I perfected my narrative by avoiding 'emotive' language and emphatic adjectives in case they opened me to criticisms of hysteria and 'somatic sensitivities'. I was wrong if I thought my sensitivity to judgement would abate when I moved into research. If anything, it magnified.

Out of necessity, I now talked more openly about my illness after decades of hiding my chronic illness from medical colleagues. Every presentation, discussion, and research meeting exposed my fear that the audience was judging me. Eventually, I learned to put this aside and distinguish between what was real and what was imagined. I began to see that even if there was judgement, it wasn't personal but came from ignorance and inexperience. To counter these preconceptions, empirical evidence must be explored, examined, collated, and disseminated before attitudes could change. While I understood there would still be scepticism, I decided I would not allow myself to be distracted by criticism but instead attend to the work required to bring forth the evidence. This pilgrimage I was now on would be long and arduous and I needed to direct my efforts towards what was changeable rather than what was beyond my control.

2.2   The Language of Experience

Hypothesis, my dear young friend, establishes itself by a cumulative process: or to use popular language, if you make the same guess often enough it ceases to be a guess and becomes a Scientific Fact. (*C.S. Lewis, The Pilgrim's Regress*)

The lived experience of chronic ill health provides a useful tool to intuit a flawed hypothesis. This became apparent during a conversation with an experienced scientific journalist interviewing me at a conference in the USA in 2022. He was writing a story on what was now being called Long COVID-19 and was interested in the research we were doing. He referred to a lecture about this condition given at a cardiac conference he had attended where it was suggested that Long COVID was purely a result of physical deconditioning. I later heard similar sentiments expressed in various other lectures. Esteemed clinicians stood in front of audiences, predominantly of other clinicians, telling them that we should "stop talking" about Long Covid lest we "put ideas" in patients' heads. To me, it was an untenable assertion that so many in society had such fragile minds that they succumbed to the mere suggestion of illness. This did not accord with my experience with real people. Rather I saw resilience and determination in most of my clinical encounters. People who were facing unimaginable suffering by all objective measures showed extraordinary braveness. To have a conscious awareness of our mortality is also to have a deep yearning to survive and thrive. This is the essence of being human. I found it inconceivable that so many were willing to withdraw from life for no other reason than a lack of will. This explanation didn't fit with my lived experience and observations.

I was preparing to provide the journalist with my thoughts on this matter when he continued. 'But this isn't the experience of the patients. **When I talk to them, I hear the same stories and patterns**. These people weren't previously in bed for days or weeks on end. Many were athletes before they got COVID-19 and despite their best efforts, months later they remain unwell'. I considered the freshness of his summation. His wasn't a naive reflection but rather an absence of encultured doctrine about illness. He didn't have an entrenched perception that these patients were the obstacles to their own healing. Instead, he believed their experience and took their story for what it was. The lived experience. The truth.

These experiences reinforced my realisation of the importance of the patient researcher paradigm. The patient experience and the interpretation of repeated patterns of manifested symptoms are more easily identifiable for researchers when patients' experiences are allowed a voice. I increasingly found confidence in my role as a conduit and interpreter of these experiences. I was able to speak the language and translate the story for research. My study participants opened up to me, comforted by the knowledge that I was not there to judge them but to understand their experiences. I could see this benefit in my research, but more importantly, as a clinician helping others live with the same illness that I had endured for nearly 30 years. I now had the ultimate pragmatic combination of scientific training, clinical relevance, and personal lived experience.

2.3   Return to the Hippocratic Way

> Once the clinical climate begins to more accurately reflect the epistemic status of medical knowledge and medical science, the way is clear for patients to become participants in designing their own treatment regimens and monitoring their own outcomes without the confounding issues of "doing the best for the patient" and "correct treatment" lurking around with an overly inflated epistemic warrant. The Hippocratics seem, of necessity perhaps, to have followed this open and exploratory approach, and any researcher who does not avail him or herself of this rich source of truly Hippocratic data is cutting off the branch on which advances in medicine have grown for over 2000 years. (Gillett 2004)

Unsurprisingly, the negative medical experiences I had 30 years ago are still commonly reported by many patients with 'invisible' illnesses today. I have long pondered why chronic and usually invisible illnesses, are subject to such apparent prejudice in medicine. My experience in research has led me to the conclusion that prejudices rarely develop from a singular cause. Rather, well-intentioned but misguided attempts to develop efficient models of research and medicine resulted in the generational exploration of disease states while ignoring the *actual experience* that resulted from these diseases. Out-dated and unexamined gender prejudices further biased interpretations of the manifestations of these illnesses. Simplistic adoption of a "one issue at a time" diagnosis and treatment model is common, despite its inadequacy in understanding and treating patients presenting with complex inter-related medical conditions. Those that did not conform to the narrative of what 'belongs' to the model were relegated to the nomenclature of 'non-organic'. Labels of 'hysteria', 'anxiety', and 'psychosomatic' were birthed, resulting in the dichotomising of the complex organism that is a human being. The dichotomy, in this instance, lay between what was deemed treatable and what was not. These misconceptions were developed into schemas that remained unexamined and were then passed down by those in positions of power and authority to generations of students who took them for gospel. Few had the time or inclination to even attempt to swim upstream against the current of dogmatised medical opinion, and those that did soon found themselves caught in the undertow and were swept briskly away.

Somewhere early in the genesis of the modern biomedical model, patients were appointed passive observers of their destinies. Concepts of disease and suffering were articulated by those without any true understanding of what that experience was. Rather than limiting bias, the medical model entrenched and cemented it. The bias of the personal experience of the patient was exchanged for that of the scientist, devoid of lived experience. It was they who hypothesised about experiences they knew nothing of and excluded symptoms that made no sense to them from concepts they explored. The biomedical model created and perpetuated a system of bias towards studying a single external element as if it were equal in importance to the vast quantity of internal and environmental factors that exert influences on the host and that likely contribute to the manifestation of chronic and complex illness; Something that rarely benefits the furthering of understanding of heterogeneous aetiologies that cause debilitating systemic syndromes such as POTS.

When we consider this in light of the pandemic, the inadequacies of the positivist medical model to fully serve our research needs are laid bare. On the one hand we should marvel at the speed with which science responded, isolated, and developed vaccines for COVID-19. This is where the biomedical model truly shines. However, this stands in stark contrast to the failings of this model in responding to the veritable wave of post-COVID-19 illness that arrived on our doorstep. Previous failings to include patients in research have left us woefully underprepared for the secondary effects of such a pandemic on society. Medicine marginalised and discredited those who experienced these conditions in relative isolation. Now that the syndromes are being experienced on a global scale we are faced with our true ignorance. We know little of what drives post-viral illnesses or how to treat them. It's not unreasonable to consider that our previous reliance on the positivist methodology "has impeded innovation in health research" that arguably could have provided answers and solutions decades before SARS-CoV-2 swept the world (Dean 2004). It's time to change the research model and re-insert the voice of the consumer experience into the hypotheses we develop. Who better to champion this cause than the researcher with lived experience?

References

Dean K. The role of methods in maintaining orthodox beliefs in health research. Soc Sci Med. 2004;58:675–85.
Gillett G. Clinical medicine and the quest for certainty. Soc Sci Med. 2004;58:727–38.

Malfait F, Francomano C, Byers P, Belmont J, Berglund B, Black J, Bloom L, Bowen JM, Brady AF, Burrows NP, Castori M, Cohen H, Colombi M, Demirdas S, de Backer J, de Paepe A, Fournel-Gigleux S, Frank M, Ghali N, Giunta C, Grahame R, Hakim A, Jeunemaitre X, Johnson D, Juul-Kristensen B, Kapferer-Seebacher I, Kazkaz H, Kosho T, Lavallee ME, Levy H, Mendoza-Londono R, Pepin M, Pope FM, Reinstein E, Robert L, Rohrbach M, Sanders L, Sobey GJ, van Damme T, Vandersteen A, Van Mourik C, Voermans N, Wheeldon N, Zschocke J, Tinkle B. The 2017 international classification of the Ehlers–Danlos syndromes. Am J Med Genet Part C Semin Med Genet. 2017;175:8–26.

Samulowitz A, Gremyr I, Eriksson E, Hensing G. "Brave men" and "emotional women": a theory-guided literature review on gender bias in health care and gendered norms towards patients with chronic pain. Pain Res Manag. 2018;2018:6358624.

Smith N. The rationality of science. Rev Métaphys Morale. 1986;91:267–70.

Wells R, Spurrier AJ, Linz D, Gallagher C, Mahajan R, Sanders P, Page A, Lau DH. Postural tachycardia syndrome: current perspectives. Vasc Health Risk Manag. 2017;14:1–11.

Who Punched Me in the Back? Becoming a CKD Researcher

Selena Firmin

Abstract Chronic kidney disease (CKD) is a silent, deadly killer. CKD causes your kidneys to become damaged and can no longer clean your blood. As a result, your body becomes overloaded with fluid, and you suffer from headaches, migraines, nausea, vomiting, and most days, it feels like someone punched you in the back, amongst other symptoms. Like many other Australians, it was too late when I was diagnosed with CKD. My kidney function had reduced to 18%. Despite following a strict diet and medication schedule, within 2 years of diagnosis, my kidney function reduced to less than 5%, and I became a haemodialysis patient. I have survived this time by using a positive mindset and regular meditation. This chapter is my story of CKD from a young child to the current day and how becoming a haemodialysis patient inspired me to become a CKD researcher with lived experience.

Keywords Chronic kidney disease · CKD · Kidney reflux disease · Nephropathy · Haemodialysis

1 Introduction

According to the Australian Institute of Health and Welfare (2023), 11% of Australians over 18 years old have signs of chronic kidney disease (CKD). CKD is when your kidneys become damaged and cannot clean your body's blood as they should (Australian Institute of Health and Welfare 2023). CKD is a growing health problem in Australia and is deadly due to its silence, showing no symptoms until its later stages when it is considered too late. This is my story of CKD, from when I was a child of ten to the current day. I discuss the physical and emotional symptoms I experience and outline some take-home messages for anyone with CKD or a loved one with CKD.

S. Firmin (✉)
Institute of Innovation, Science and Sustainability, Federation University,
Ballarat, VIC, Australia
e-mail: s.firmin@federation.edu.au

© The Author(s), under exclusive license to Springer Nature Singapore Pte Ltd. 2024
A. Stranieri et al. (eds.), *Research Partners with Lived Experience*,
https://doi.org/10.1007/978-981-97-0033-2_2

2   CKD Journey

It was 1978 in Australia, a time of disco, bell-bottom pants, cheese fondue and the Ford Cortina. I was in grade 5 and had turned 10 years old. I was a happy, carefree little kid. I had a loving, supportive family. I loved horses, swimming, and reading. My world was about to change.

3   Ten Years Old

One morning I woke up with a sharp burning pain in my middle to lower back on the left-hand side. It felt like someone had repeatedly punched me. Over the coming months, this pain became my constant companion and along with it, fever, vomiting, headaches, and a burning pain when passing urine. I now know these were urinary tract infections (UTIs). A UTI is a bacterial infection that can affect your urethra, bladder, or kidneys (Kidney Health Australia 2020a). UTIs can cause pain when urinating and are embarrassing as you feel you must urinate frequently.

I was hospitalised on and off for over 12 months and subjected to many medical tests before a local general practitioner (GP) determined that I had kidney reflux disease, also known as reflux nephropathy. Kidney reflux disease is caused by the backflow of urine from your bladder up the ureters into your kidney (Kidney Health Australia 2020a). Suppose you can imagine a hose with a kink in it. The water flows backward. My left-hand side ureter was like a hose with a kink. I later discovered this condition was genetic, which means it was likely inherited from my parents, most likely my dad, as my paternal grandmother died of bowel cancer. My paternal cousin has Crohn's disease, and my father and his sister both have colonoscopies every 12 months due to polyps requiring removal. Perhaps there is a link between all these maladies? I don't know, but that is my aunt's theory. The kink in my ureter was fixed through surgery. The surgeons were able to straighten it. This was followed by 12 months of bacterium taken orally. Bacterium is a strong medication that is a combination of two antibiotics. I recall it was a pink colour and tasted awful. It was 10 years before I experienced these symptoms again.

4   Twenty Years Old

I was 20 years old and working full-time in my second year of working post-secondary school. My symptoms were the same as those I experienced when I was ten, the burning pain in my middle to lower back on the left-hand side, along with fever, vomiting, and headaches. I attended the same GP clinic, and they had my history on file. The doctor had said I was experiencing UTIs. I was hospitalised and had surgery. However, the kink in my ureter had not reappeared. I took antibiotics, the infection cleared up, and my medical team sought no further medical interventions. In retrospect, if I had only known, this was a massive warning sign that something was wrong.

At 22 years old, after 4 years of working, I returned to study, completing a Bachelor of Computing. I had to study it part-time so I could support myself. I spent most of my money on a car and a horse-riding habit. So I did as many night classes as possible and worked during the daytime. However, it still took me 5 years to complete the degree. I didn't think much about research during this time, but I always enjoyed researching for papers and assignments. I worked as a database programmer for 4 years after completing my degree. By the time I was 30, I had started as a full-time multimedia and web development TAFE teacher. I also returned to study and completed a Graduate Certificate in Education (Tertiary Education) and a Diploma of Vocational Education and Training. The Graduate Certificate in Education (Tertiary Education) was my first introduction to formal research. As part of the assessment in this course, I was required to write my first literature review. My topic was using the Internet as a delivery strategy for learning and teaching. This was the start of my passion for finding ways to improve my students' learning experiences through research. During this time, my daughter was born. She was a great baby, and I managed my work, study, and family duties by getting up early in the morning.

5 Mid-30s

By my mid-30s, I had started experiencing symptoms of chronic kidney disease, although I did not realise it then. These symptoms included UTIs, frequent urine output, lethargy, chronic headaches, insomnia, and feelings of sadness leading to depression.

I tried homeopathic remedies such as St. Johns Wart and Vitamin B to improve my general feeling of wellness, and these did help. I also took Valerian tablets to help me sleep, but I had mixed success with these.

I visited my GP regarding my chronic headaches. My GP recommend I take Panadol and Ibuprofen. At the time, I did not know it, but I later discovered that anyone with decreased kidney function should avoid Ibuprofen. Ibuprofen restricts blood flow in your arteries, veins, and kidneys to lessen pain and swelling. The decreased blood flow can reduce kidney function and increase the risk of your kidneys failing (Cheong 2022). While the Panadol and Ibuprofen alleviated some of the headache pain, they did not fix it completely. By then, I had started to get regular migraines. Migraines are also a symptom of CKD. Migraines are a severe form of headache, with symptoms including extreme throbbing pain, nausea, vomiting, and light sensitivity. I experienced all these symptoms and still had no cure.

A friend suggested I get my eyes tested. As a daily computer user, this might be part of my problem. Therefore, I visited an optometrist who diagnosed me with long- and short-sightedness. A person with long-sightedness (hypermetropia) cannot see near objects, and a person with short-sightedness (myopia) cannot see distant objects (Department of Health 2021). The optometrist told me the use of glasses would fix my headaches. Unfortunately, these did not improve my headaches, but I could see better (laughing).

Then I tried an acupuncturist. Acupuncturists use small sterile, disposable needles to penetrate your skin to activate points of healing through gentle and specific flicks of the needles (Australian Government 2021). Acupuncture is known to help with headaches and migraines. Unfortunately, it did not work for me.

I also tried deep tissue massage, reiki, myotherapy, physiotherapy, and chiropractic care. Chiropractors treat back pain and issues with the musculoskeletal system (Allied Health Professions Australia 2023). Regular visits to a chiropractor did not eliminate my headaches and migraines, but we did manage to get them somewhat under control.

I also started using meditation to control the migraine pain. Meditation is a technique where you focus and train your mind to achieve a clear and emotionally calm state (Walsh and Shapiro 2006). At the time, I did not know how valuable this technique would be in managing pain and depressive feelings.

I took on a managerial role at the TAFE institution, which amalgamated with the local university. I studied for a Master of Business Administration (MBA) for 12 months. However, after being offered a lecturing position in the university's higher education division, I transferred to a computing honours program. Honours were my introduction to data collection, thesis writing and paper publication. My honours research project continued my passion for improving student learning experiences by examining varying degrees of computer-mediated communication use by IT students. During this time, my son was born. I used to take him to my classes with me. He never cried; it was like he knew he had to be good. I commenced a part-time PhD in Computer Science at the end of my honour's degree. My topic examined the role of technology in shaping IT academics' pedagogy. I loved the research but found it challenging to balance it with family commitments, teaching, and administration.

6   Mid to Late 40s

By my mid-40s, I was also experiencing significant weight gain, which was partly due to getting older, but also, I did not realise that I had considerable water retention, known as hypervolemia. Hypervolemia or fluid overload is when you have too much water in your body (Cirion 2017). A reduction in the function of my kidneys caused fluid overload. The fluid overload also caused other symptoms, including shortness of breath, high blood pressure (or hypertension), delayed wound healing, and other health problems.

I tried many diets to lose weight without much success. I visited the local GP, who said he would provide me with appetite suppressant drugs if I could lose 5 kg. After months of unsuccessfully trying, I returned to the local GP, a new doctor. This doctor said, "You need to lose weight. Get a personal trainer". I felt a bit upset because I had been trying. However, I rallied and joined a gym but continued to put on weight, and the shortness of breath became so bad I could barely walk. I went to the doctor again, and he gave me a Ventolin puffer. The Ventolin puffer failed to work, so I started my research, and I found Ventolin puffers to be useful if you cannot get the air out of your lungs. My problem was the opposite. I could not get enough air into my lungs.

My left leg swelled up and changed colour. It looked like a giant hot dog (laughing). I was also unable to keep any food down and was constantly vomiting. So my husband took me to the local hospital, where they admitted me and did some blood tests. They also gave me some penicillin. I was allergic to penicillin, causing swelling and red welts all over my body. They discharged me and told me to go to the nearest major hospital, about an hour's drive away. I discovered that being unable to be transferred easily was one of the many shortcomings of the public hospital system. I ended up being in the hospital for 6 weeks.

I was sent to a metropolitan hospital for a kidney biopsy in the third week. This was when we discovered I had stage 4 kidney disease, and my kidney function was down to 18%. A normal 50-year-old person has a kidney function of approximately 75%. The kidney biopsy was brutal. A radiologist carried out the procedure. He used what looked like a large knitting needle to take a sample of my left kidney. He told me he would need to take two samples, but he missed one and had to take three samples (ouch). The procedure was rescheduled three times because my blood pressure was too high, and I ended up fasting for 4 days. The fourth time they used a clonidine transdermal (skin patch) to control my high blood pressure. I recall asking the nurse to cover me up because I felt embarrassed when I was left on the operation table with nothing on. When I left the operation, my mum was crying in the waiting room. This devastated me. Up to this point, I had been quite stoic, but when I saw my mum upset, I had an epiphany and knew that even though I was an adult, she still loved me as much as I love my children. I could not stand the thought of my parents being so upset and taking on the burden of my illness.

I had regular appointments with the nephrologist and the kidney dietician specialist in the following months. A nephrologist is a medical doctor specialising in kidney care (Cleveland Clinic 2023). I also started to read a lot of literature to develop a better understanding of my disease.

7 Early 50s

Two months after my 50th birthday, I was diagnosed with stage 5 kidney disease, and my kidney function had dropped to less than 5%. I started haemodialysis. Without dialysis my body would have shut down and I would passed away in about 10 days. According to Kidney Health Australia (2020b) "haemodialysis is the treatment for kidney failure. Your blood is pumped through special tubing to a haemodialysis machine. The machine acts like a kidney, filtering waste products from your blood before returning it to your body". I was given a permacath to administer my dialysis. A permacath or haemodialysis catheter is a set of plastic tubes typically positioned into the blood vessel in your neck or upper chest on the right side of your heart (Tasmanian Government 2022). The red tube takes your blood to the dialysis machine for cleaning and fluid removal, while the blue tube returns the blood to the patient. The treatment typically lasts 4 hours, three times a week, however, you need to arrive at the dialysis ward at least half an hour before your start time, and it takes another half an hour to get unhooked from the machine, so overall, it takes a good 5 hours.

In the meantime, I went to a vascular surgeon (a surgeon who treats diseases of blood vessels, arteries and veins) to have a fistula made. To create a fistula, the vascular surgeon joined an artery to a vein making super blood flow. When you rest your hand on the join site (called a bruit pronounced brew-ee) you can feel a strong buzz sensation. The buzz sensation decreases as you get further away from the bruit site. My fistula was created on my inside lower left arm as they avoid your dominant arm. A fistula takes about 3 months to mature before it can be used.

Like many other CKD patients, my permacath became infected with golden staph (staphylococcus aureus) despite a meticulous and regimented care routine. They removed the permacath, and I ended up with three more permacaths before my fistula was ready. After researching, I discovered haemodialysis patients are particularly susceptible to staphylococcal bacteria. Staphylococcus aureus is a common bacterial infection that causes skin infections and serious infections like septicaemia (blood poisoning) and pneumonia (Vandecasteele et al. 2009). I had the more serious type of blood poisoning, golden staph, with a high fever and shortness of breath. It took around 6 months to get diagnosed. At first, I suffered from back pain, nausea, headaches, and a low-grade temperature. Over a 6-month period, my family called an ambulance at least three times, and they took me to the emergency department (ED) and the GP multiple times. One of the times, we arrived at the ED to find out my husband had taken us to the wrong hospital. He was beside himself. My then 16-year-old son bravely pushed me up the street to the private hospital in a wheelchair. I was admitted and was given eight blood transfusions. I still think about all the wonderful people who donated the blood that saved my life. I am forever grateful. Also, thank you to my son. No 16-year-old should have to do what he did that night.

Eventually, I could no longer walk and was in a wheelchair experiencing frequent electric-like shocks down my legs. My daughter took me to the GP, who was very concerned and phoned my nephrologist, and both agreed I needed to go to the ED immediately. My daughter took me, and the ED doctor ordered an MRI. The MRI revealed I had golden staph in two vertebrae of my middle back. I was immediately transported by ambulance to a large metropolitan hospital, where a neurosurgeon (a surgeon who treats disorders of the brain, spine and nerves) conducted a laminectomy. The surgeon removed two infected vertebrae and cleaned out the site removing the pressure on my spinal cord, which was causing the electric shocks. It was my 51st birthday, the day after my spine surgery. That was the loneliest birthday I had ever had. I felt trapped in a hospital bed, hundreds of kilometres away from the love and support of my friends and family. My mum sent me some flowers that never got to me, and I like to think that someone deserving got those. After that, I worked hard to keep a positive mindset, and my meditation practices helped me deal with the pain.

After 2 weeks, I was transported back to the hospital in my new hometown. After a couple of days, when I checked my fistula's bruit, I discovered there was no buzz. They sent me back to the big city hospital, where I had an operation to dislodge a blood clot that had blocked my fistula. Ugggh, what a horrible experience. They give you a sedative, so you are awake through the operation, then inject some medication which hopefully dissolves the clot. Unfortunately, it did not work, so they inserted a balloon device, pumped air into it, and managed to dislodge the clot. I was very lucky. They returned me to my new hometown hospital, and I was admitted for about another 6 months, most of that was in the rehab ward.

After 6 months, my neurosurgeon ordered a CT scan and an MRI. I slowly walked into my appointment using a walking frame with my daughter and her partner. My daughter was an angel, taking on parental duties for her brother, dropping him off to football training, cooking tea, doing the laundry and looking after all my needs. The neurosurgeon was a registrar. He showed us pictures taken by the MRI. You can see a bend in my spinal cord. See Fig. 1. His eyes filled with tears as he told us he expected I would never walk again. We had not realised there was a danger of paralysis. Every 6 months after this, I have an MRI and CT scan. I still

Fig. 1 MRI of the thoracic spine

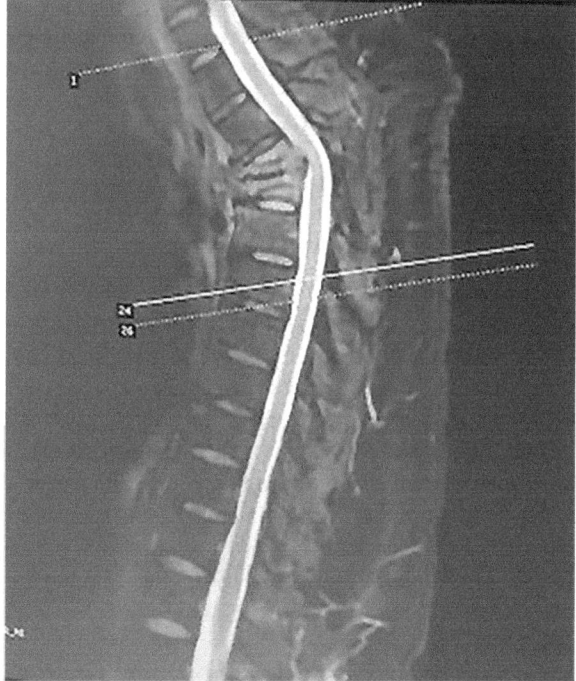

have these scans so the neurosurgeons can monitor the health of my spinal cord. The neurosurgeons had decided to do a second operation to stabilise my spine a couple of years ago. However, the second operation was cancelled due to COVID-19. The operation would have taken about 6 hours, as they had to deflate a lung and create a cadge out of donor's bone to fit around the spinal cord. I did not have the second operation as the neurosurgeon felt my spine had stabilised itself over time.

The saddest part of all this for me was no more horse riding. I had horses since I was 12 years old. I still had horse riding dreams and had to take these off my bucket list. I had three horses at the time. One we gave to a lovely lady, another we had to send to heaven because he had turned blind, and the third beautiful pony still lives on the property that we sold. The new owner was happy to keep her there. I still dream of bringing her to my new home, as we have room for her here, but I no longer have the energy to look after her. This is perhaps the worse symptom of CKD— lethargy. Sometimes your body feels like lead, and you can hardly move one leg in front of another. Other times if you overdrink, you feel like a balloon full of water that is so full it is about to burst.

After the operation, my family moved to a rental property in what I call my new hometown. This town had a public hospital with a dialysis unit. My son had to change schools and leave all his friends. To say we were devastated would be an understatement. My daughter was at university, and the address change worked well for her. I had to sell my horse float to pay the rent, and my husband was left to renovate and clean our 100-year-old house. The guilt I felt and still feel is overwhelming. My husband lived in that town his whole life. The town was so grateful for all the community work he had done over the years, receiving an Australia Day award, and they threw a going-away party for him, naming the football rooms after him. Luckily, we sold our house after just 1 week on the market. We purchased a new home which everyone loves. After about 6 weeks, I returned to work 0.8, taking 1 day a week as sick leave.

8   Health Informatics Research

I started reading as many kidney and haemodialysis research papers as I could get my hands on to gain a better understanding of my condition. I was also kindly introduced to a wonderful, selfless woman who builds Apps for the chronically ill in her own time. We developed a project proposal and submitted several grant applications to build an all-inclusive App for haemodialysis patients. Unfortunately, we were unsuccessful with the grant applications. However, we published a research-in-progress paper at the Health Informatics and Knowledge Management (HIKM.org) conference. The paper's purpose was to present an approach to understanding the critical challenges the chronically ill face, including those suffering from heart disease, diabetes, and CKD. Then use those critical challenges to inform the design of a customised app for patient self-management (Khurrum and Firmin 2022). We have been invited to extend the paper into a journal article and will look at doing that. Since then, we have searched for a potential PhD student to develop and test the App we want to build. As part of the same project, we are writing a systematic literature review paper comparing Apps and their shortcoming for haemodialysis patients.

At the same time, several colleagues successfully applied for several small health informatics grants. We used the grant money to purchase Fitbit watches and used a trial version of an app built by an industry partner that sends do's (positive affirmations) to a small group of haemodialysis patients. I participated in the trial and found the positive affirmations helped boost my motivation and confidence in dealing with my condition. Other patients also expressed the inspiration and enthusiasm gained through receiving the positive affirmations. We also published a research-in-progress paper outlining our Fitbit project at the HIKM conference. The second health informatics grant project is still underway and is an extension of the Fitbit project.

While my research in this area is still in its infancy, I plan to continue this work and help as many haemodialysis patients as possible.

9   Fifty-Five Plus

As the damage to my kidneys cannot be reversed, my goal is to get a kidney transplant. When the nephrologist told me the average life expectancy for a haemodialysis patient is 10 years, I was shocked. However, after some research, I discovered this is an average figure. Most haemodialysis patients are older, which skews the figures. According to the Australian Institute of Health and Welfare (2023), approximately 45% of all CKD patients are 75+ years, while in my age group, 55–64 years, the rate is approximately 10%.

When I get my transplant, a donor kidney from a living or deceased person will be placed in my left-hand side lower abdomen. The operation will take about 4 hours, and I will be in hospital for about a week. If I am lucky enough to get a deceased donated kidney, it may take a couple of weeks to start working, so I may have to continue dialysis for that time. My other kidneys will be left where they are unless they cause other medical issues. I will have to take immunosuppressants (medicine to stop my body from rejecting the new kidney) for the remainder of my life (National Kidney Foundation 2023). According to the Harvard Medical School Teaching Hospital (2022), if I get a living donor kidney, it will last approximately 12–20 years. If I get a deceased kidney donor, it will last approximately 8–12 years. Either way, I will live longer if I am lucky enough to get a kidney transplant.

10 Concluding Remarks

My take-home messages for anyone with CKD or if you have a loved one with CKD are to keep working, exercise gently, and negotiate with your loved ones how much you can do around the house because you won't be able to do what you used to. Take your medication, stick to the diet and fluid restrictions and, importantly, be proactive with your health care. I can't stress this enough if you are unwell or unsatisfied with your doctor's diagnosis, get second opinions and research the illness yourself. As a patient, you must be proactive, self-aware and understand your condition. Use meditation to control your pain, stay positive, keep a positive mindset, and be grateful daily.

References

Allied Health Professions Australia. Chiropractic. 2023. Available https://ahpa.com.au/allied-health-professions/chiropractic/. Accessed 18 January.

Australian Government. Acupuncture. 2021. Available https://www.healthdirect.gov.au/acupuncture. Accessed 18 January.

Australian Institute of Health and Welfare. Chronic kidney disease. 2023. Available https://www.aihw.gov.au/reports-data/health-conditions-disability-deaths/chronic-kidney-disease/overview. Accessed 20 May 2023.

Cheong J. Does Ibuprofen affect your kidneys? 2022. Available https://healthmatch.io/kidney-disease/is-ibuprofen-bad-for-your-kidneys. Accessed 18 January 2023.

Cirion E. Hypervolemia (fluid overload). 2017. Available https://www.healthline.com/health/hypervolemia. Accessed 18 January 2023.

Cleveland Clinic. 2023. Nephrologist. Available https://my.clevelandclinic.org/health/articles/24214-nephrologist. Accessed 26 April 2023.

Department of Health. Eyes. 2021. Available https://www.betterhealth.vic.gov.au/conditionsandtreatments/eyes. Accessed 18 January 2023.

Firmin S, Khurram S. 2022. Informing App Design to Reduce Self-Management Challenges Identified for Chronic Disease. In Australasian Computer Science Week. 2022:246–9.

Harvard Medical School Teaching Hospital. The benefits of kidney transplant versus dialysis. 2022. Accessed 18 May 2022.

Kidney Health Australia. Urinary tract infections (UTI)s. 2020a. Available https://kidney.org.au/your-kidneys/what-is-kidney-disease/types-of-kidney-disease/utis. Accessed 22 February 2020.

Kidney Health Australia. Your kidneys. 2020b. Available https://kidney.org.au/your-kidneys/know-your-kidneys/. Accessed: 28 April 2020.

National Kidney Foundation. Kidney transplant. 2023. Available https://www.kidney.org/atoz/content/kidney-transplant#who-can-get-kidney-transplant. Accessed 20 May 2023.

Tasmanian Government. Understanding your haemodialysis catheter (permacath). 2022. Available https://www.health.tas.gov.au/health-topics/kidney-renal/kidney-treatments/understanding-your-haemodialysis-catheter-permacath. Accessed 22 February 2022.

Vandecasteele S, Boelaert J, De Vriese A. Staphylococcus aureus infections in hemodialysis: what a nephrologist should know. Clin J Am Soc Nephrol. 2009;4(8):1388–400.

Walsh R, Shapiro SL. The meeting of meditative disciplines and western psychology: a mutually enriching dialogue. Am Psychol. 2006;61(3):227–39.

Zebras Have Spots

Karen Raymond

Abstract This is the story of a woman born with a rare, genetic, autoinflammatory disease that was a life-limiting mystery until she was finally diagnosed at the age of 43. Her diagnosis of familial cold autoinflammatory syndrome (one of three cryopyrin-associated periodic syndromes) only came following information provided by another family member. Continued post-diagnosis frustration with medical practitioners motivated her to complete a Bachelor of Science (Biomedical Science) and immerse herself in the research of NLRP3, the gene responsible for her lifelong private struggle. NLRP3 has been implicated in many more common diseases and here the author describes her particular battle with inflammatory bowel disease, wondering aloud whether it is part of her primary condition. This informative story is told with candour and shades of dark humour, giving the reader a front-row seat to life with a rare disease in Australia.

Keywords NLRP3 inflammasome autoinflammatory cryopyrin colitis IBD

1 Introduction

I was born sick, but there was nothing wrong with me. From birth I had painful, red, hot, skin rashes that didn't respond to antihistamines, occasional joint swelling that looked like but definitely wasn't arthritis, occasional foot swelling that looked like but definitely wasn't gout, occasional pink eye that looked like but definitely wasn't conjunctivitis (Fig. 1). I had migraines that were obviously caused by something I was eating. I had chronic low iron anaemia because of something I wasn't eating. My inflammation markers were always only marginally elevated so I was probably always getting over an infection. I started to bleed from my backside and suffer

K. Raymond (✉)
The University of Adelaide, Adelaide, SA, Australia
e-mail: karen@pazray.com.au

A. Stranieri et al. (eds.), *Research Partners with Lived Experience*,
https://doi.org/10.1007/978-981-97-0033-2_3

27

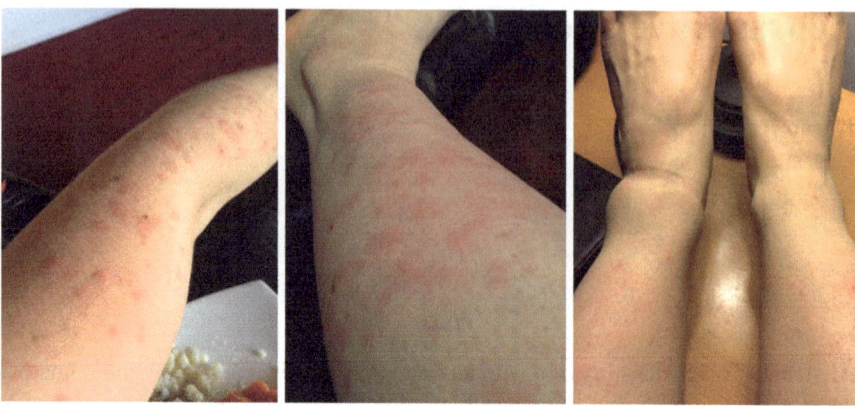

Fig. 1 My CAPS rash, arm and leg. My CAPS swollen ankle joint

fatigue to the point of being upright for barely 2 h a day, but all that was probably because I had an underlying anxiety disorder and was not managing my stress.

Actually, I had a rare, genetic disorder that probably never would have been diagnosed if some doctors in Melbourne weren't interested in patient stories. Thanks to them diagnosing my second cousin, I eventually found out what I had and could take the diagnosis to my doctors and start treatment. Thankfully, I had a contrary and negative specialist who was resistant to my questions and dismissive of the ideas I would share from research I had been reading. The gaslighting motivated me to get an undergraduate degree in biomedical science, to learn the language of researchers and properly understand how my disease worked.

The name of my condition is cryopyrin-associated periodic syndrome (CAPS). It is a rare, autoinflammatory syndrome caused by gain of function mutations in the NLRP3 gene, a cytosolic receptor in the innate immune system most famous for nucleating the NLRP3 inflammasome. There are three different flavours of CAPS that fall on a spectrum of severity (Booshehri and Hoffman 2019):

Familial cold autoinflammatory syndrome (FCAS) is considered to be the mildest form, with systemic symptoms triggered by generalised exposure to cold, described in the literature as neutrophilic rash, headache, conjunctivitis, arthralgia, occasional swollen joints and fever.

Muckle-Wells syndrome (MWS) is the intermediate condition that has all the FCAS symptoms with more frequency and extra triggers like heat and stress, plus sensorineural hearing loss, migraines, gastrointestinal involvement and an increased risk of developing secondary amyloidosis, particularly if untreated.

The most severe form has two names, neonatal-onset multisystem inflammatory disease (NOMID) which is used more in the USA, and chronic infantile neurological cutaneous and articular (CINCA) disease, favoured in Europe. NOMID/CINCA is more likely than the other two forms to be diagnosed early because of its severity and developmental effects. This disease has the features of the first two, but headaches and migraines are now aseptic meningitis, with extra physical features such as bony overgrowth, particularly in the knees, frontal bossing, the technical term for big forehead and intellectual disability. Without treatment, children with NOMID/CINCA will often not reach adulthood.

As CAPS is one of a growing number of emerging autoinflammatory diseases (please look them up, they are fascinating), there has been a push to standardise the nomenclature to indicate the nature of the disease as autoinflammatory and the gene involved. I'm not sure who ultimately decided that autoinflammatory diseases should be termed AIDs but I'm not sure NLRP3-AID (mild), NLRP3-AID (moderate) and NLRP3-AID (severe) are going to catch on with patients. Many of us with CAPS don't fit neatly in any one box. Others are clinically diagnosed and respond well to treatment but no mutation is found in the NLRP3 gene.

The mutation I have in my NLRP3 gene is A439V and it has been described in the literature as both FCAS and MWS, which is not wrong. I am part of a large, Australian family group with this mutation and we are all over the spectrum. My phenotype best fits the description of MWS minus the hearing loss.

2   Back Story of Life with CAPS

Living with CAPS is like living with arms. You know you have them, you're aware of them all the time, they're just part of you. You don't know what it's like not to have them. It's your normal. My normal was waking up and doing a full body scan to see if anything had popped up overnight, like swollen feet or ankles, a painful red eye, a migraine or any leftover rash from the day before, if it had been a particularly bad one. From there it was a matter of surviving whatever I had to do that day before I could get home and into a hot bath, keeping warm and staying horizontal for the rest of the evening. When I felt up to it there was a particular step aerobics class I used to enjoy at my gym on a Wednesday, but I'd be rotten afterwards, full shut down. What the hell is full shut down? Sorry, it's my normal so I forget people don't know what I mean. Let me paint you a picture of a full shut down.

> My whole body, covered with rash, begins to ache, just slightly at first, like a tidal wave coming in from a distance and from experience I know it's going to be bad… then it gets worse and worse, the aching pain rolling in with unstoppable force. (Doctors would ask, 'Where do you get pain?' I would answer, 'Everywhere'. They'd press me for specifics. I'd say, 'Everywhere I have skin'. Their sceptical frown became known as 'that look'.) The pain is in my skin and all my tissues. I get cold to my core and can't get warm. I want to sit right in a fire. The closest thing I have is a hot bath. I try to make the transition from bath to pyjamas without getting cold. The heat lamps are on (radiant heat is always best), the towel is dry and right where I can grab it. Getting out hurts. I dry myself and get to bed as quickly as I can, clutching what I lovingly refer to as my chuck bucket, as nausea features. I shiver and shake and my body goes into spasms, rigors. I use every mindfulness technique in the book to stay calm, breathe and relax. If I can just fall asleep it will all be over. Until tomorrow.

I met Paul in 1993 at the Flinders University gym. I was doing a perfunctory Bachelor of Arts just to prove I could; Paul lived around the corner and got free access because his mate worked on the desk. One of the first things we did was go on a ski trip. It seems crazy now, but I had been on ski trips through school and been more or less okay. On the first night, I had a full shut down episode. Can you imagine? You've just met the girl of your dreams and, as the sun goes down she's covered in a rash and having some kind of seizure. A lesser man would have run for his life. Luckily for me, Paul is a practical kind of guy. He went and collected every blanket in the establishment and piled them up on me like some kind of reverse princess and the pea. That's the kind of guy Paul is. We got married and had a carpet cleaning business that we ran together for 20 years. Did you think I would say we got married and had kids? We didn't have kids. I didn't know what was wrong with me but I knew my Dad had it and I knew my Grandma had it. I didn't know what a gene was but I didn't need a science degree to know I had an inherited condition. Plus, I didn't have the energy to take care of kids. As the years went by I became more certain I'd made the right decision on that front. My health was slowly getting worse and my world was getting smaller. In 2014 I got whooping cough (confirmed *Bordetella parapertussis*) thanks to the hero complex of an idiot at my gym, and that's when the bum bleeding started. Not huge amounts, but it was there. And I was always backed up. You might think, 'Ah, she's probably just got a haemorrhoid from straining.' That's what one gastroenterologist wrote to my GP, without bothering to look, after diagnosing me with ulcerative proctitis.

You might also think, 'Gross, I don't want to hear this.' Get used to it if you're going into medicine. Bodies are gross. But I've never had a haemorrhoid in my life. I was using all my mindfulness techniques to keep calm and look after my butthole, which I knew was in trouble. After the gastroenterologist wrote to my GP also suggesting I had an underlying anxiety disorder, I moved on to a general physician (I had shown the gastroenterologist the rash on my arms and asked him if he thought that was anxiety) who decided I was just a stressed person who needed to restructure my daily activities so as not to over-exhaust myself. I couldn't have been clearer with him when I said I do not have stress in my life. No kids, a wonderfully supportive husband (Fig. 2), a wonderfully supportive family, a successful business that

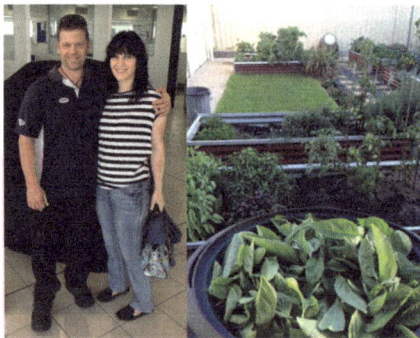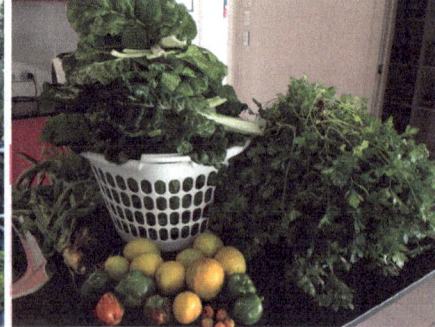

Fig. 2 Looking great but feeling awful. Me (left) with my husband, our veggie garden and a fresh harvest of home-grown produce

only needed me part-time because of wonderful staff who ran it beautifully. Yoga classes, meditation, no expectations. But there was nothing wrong with me, so it must be stress.

When I first started to bleed, my GP told me to stop eating dairy. I thought that was weird because I'd never had any issue with dairy before, why would that suddenly be a problem? Ulcerative proctitis is a type of colitis, and I looked into a few eating regimens that claimed to help this type of condition. I settled on the specific carbohydrate diet (SCD) (Gottschall 1986) and for 18 months I didn't eat sugar, grain, lactose or starch. I made my own long-fermentation yoghurt, using starter cultures specifically recommended for this diet. I did not cheat even once. I grew my own veggies (still do—Fig. 2) and made all my own sauces from scratch with my Thermomix (mostly still do that too) and started making my own chicken broth. After 18 months I looked great but was sicker than ever.

I had no energy, my normal had become to get up, have breakfast with Paul (he would cook for me) and clean the kitchen. Paul would go to work and I would lie on the couch, playing on my iPad for the rest of the day because I didn't have the energy to do anything else. I would attend to any correspondence but minimally. I felt my life force was ever so slowly draining away until, out of the blue, I got an email from my Dad (Fig. 3).

As I read the information from Dad's cousin, tears ran down my face. Words can't even begin to describe the sense of relief and validation. At the same time, all hope was lost. No diet was going to fix me.

I went to see my GP who ordered genetic testing and referred me to a rheumatologist. The rheumatologist had heard of these conditions but said they were extremely rare and the chance I could have this would be like winning the lottery. She also said she needed time to read up on the condition and how to prescribe

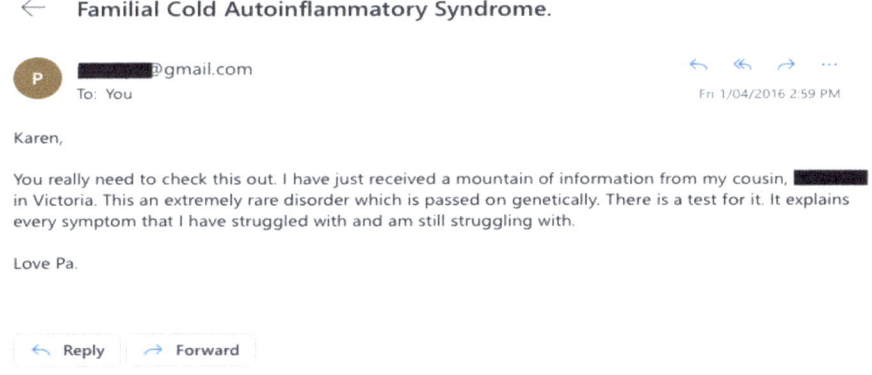

Fig. 3 Email from my father that unlocked the mystery of our lifetime

anakinra [1] or, as she wrote in her letter 'Anikera' and 'Ankera'. This person held my health in her hands! I asked how long she would need because I was desperate for treatment. She shot me a filthy look and did not answer. I asked my GP for another referral. He referred me to a rheumatologist who had at least one other FCAS patient.

When I made the appointment, I was told I would be seeing a registrar and when I looked up that registrar his interest was celiac disease. I had already been down that road and wasn't going down it again. I went to get my medical records from an immunologist's office where, 8 years earlier, I'd gone through allergy and celiac testing and been told I had 'idiopathic urticaria'. As I was driving away, the immunologist himself called me and he said he did think I probably had FCAS and, because he believed me, I asked my GP for a third referral, back to him. Incredibly, he refused to give me any treatment until genetics had confirmed the condition, despite PBS [2] rules allowing for a clinical diagnosis. All in all it took 9 weeks from Dad's email to treatment. Every day I was suffering and it felt so cruel to know there was something that could make me feel better, but I was at the mercy of doctors who were holding it just out of my reach.

3   Starting Treatment and Life After Diagnosis

The first injection of anakinra had to be done at the immunologist's office, to make sure I didn't have a reaction like anaphylaxis. Within minutes, the tide went out. I kept looking at my body and checking for pain. Paul had taken me to the doctor and was well-versed in the routine of getting me home as soon as possible but, on this day, I told him to wait. We visited a friend. After that, he again wanted to take me home and again I said, 'No wait, let's go to the beach'. He looked at me in wonder and we drove to Semaphore. We got out of the car and walked over the little sand hill to the beach. Tears began to flow. I realised I'd never expected to see the ocean or feel the sea air again in my life. I could hardly believe this drug was actually working. Suddenly I wanted to do everything immediately, before the other shoe dropped, as it always did.

It was a slow drop but, as my body became accustomed to Kineret, I began to experience break through symptoms. It was mainly in the form of waking up rough. When I say rough, I mean bad head pain, body pain and generally achy. Plus, after a record 6 weeks of remission, my bum had begun bleeding again. Seven months after starting Kineret I asked about increasing the dose. I'd joined a Facebook group for CAPS patients and seen that people were on higher doses. Apparently it was not uncommon to need a dose increase after a few months. This gave me a bit of relief

---

[1] Anakinra, brand name Kineret, is a small molecule interleukin 1 receptor antagonist, given subcutaneously. It is the only treatment available for CAPS in Australia.

[2] *PBS* pharmaceutical benefits scheme.

that the drug would continue to work, but my immunologist refused, with the reasoning, 'You have FCAS and the Kineret dose for FCAS is 100mg daily. Higher doses are simply not done'. Knowing this was flat out untrue, I protested strongly. I showed him the Australian Register of Therapeutic Goods product information for Kineret (Fig. 4) and argued that I had already tried a second shot when I'd experienced break through symptoms and it had helped.

He agreed to let me try but said he'd need some kind of clinical marker to justify it. Because I'd reminded him of the initial proctitis remission, he decided on faecal calprotectin. Faecal calprotectin measures calprotectin in your poo. Calprotectin is found inside white blood cells called neutrophils, so if you have a lot of it in your poo, it means you have a lot of debris from neutrophils and that generally means you have inflammation. A good number is below 50 μg/g. Mine was over 1200. After 3 months on two daily shots it went down to 300. Despite the improvement, he pointed out that it was still 6× higher than the cut off and remained convinced I had two different conditions. He told me it was too easy to ascribe everything to this condition and I asked him why he thought it couldn't be part of it. His answer was simply that it was a different mechanism and that was the end of it.

CAPS

Starting dose:

The recommended starting dose for both adults and children is 1-2 mg/kg/day by subcutaneous (SC) injection. The therapeutic response is primarily reflected by reduction in clinical symptoms such as fever, rash, joint pain, and headache, but also in inflammatory serum markers (CRP/SAA levels), or occurrence of flares.

KINERET® PI, vA12-0   Page 1 of 18

Maintenance dose in mild CAPS (FCAS, mild MWS):

Patients are usually well-controlled by maintaining the recommended starting dose (1-2 mg/kg/day).

Maintenance dose in severe CAPS (MWS and NOMID/CINCA):

Dose increases may become necessary within 1-2 months based on therapeutic response. The usual maintenance dose in severe CAPS is 3-4 mg/kg/day, which can be adjusted to a maximum of 8 mg/kg/day.

In addition to the evaluation of clinical symptoms and inflammatory markers in severe CAPS, assessments of inflammation of the CNS, including the inner ear (MRI or CT, lumbar puncture, and audiology) and eyes (ophthalmological assessments) are recommended after an initial 3 months of treatment, and thereafter every 6 months, until effective treatment doses have been identified. When patients are clinically well-controlled, CNS and ophthalmological monitoring may be conducted yearly.

Once daily administration is generally recommended, but the dose may be split into twice daily administrations. Each syringe is intended for a single use. A new syringe must be used for each dose. Any unused portion after each dose should be discarded.

Fig. 4 Excerpt of Kineret product information from the Australian Register of Therapeutic Goods ARTG ID 82872 http://www.ebs.tga.gov.au/ebs/picmi/picmirepository.nsf/pdf?OpenAgent=&id=CP-2021-PI-02086-1 as at 10 November 2022

Frustrated, I decided to find out what these supposed different mechanisms were exactly. Not one to do things by halves, I enrolled in a Bachelor of Science at Adelaide University, because my high school matriculation score from 1989 was not high enough for the Bachelor of Science (Biomed) that I wanted to do. I could transfer after first year if I achieved a grade point average (GPA) of 6 or higher, which meant I needed distinctions across the board. I was going to have to work super hard. I had done the Bachelor of Arts at Flinders University in the 1990s and cruised through with credits. I'd done no science, apart from maths, that I could recall since year 9 physics in 1986. I remembered getting a minus score on a test about photosynthesis for being a smart alec, which was possibly also year 9 and that was my entire recollection of biology.

4 Going to University

Going to university at the age of 44 is hard. Add to this the daily injections, abdominal pain, bum bleeding, fatigue and anxiety. University was both amazing and terrifying. I met two people at orientation day who would become my favourite study buddies. Kira was another mature-aged student, but only in her 20s and raising two young sons. Jack was a young lad straight from high school, strategically smart enough to know he'd probably get a better grade hanging out with us. At the start of my first chemistry practical (which sounds weird so practicals will hereafter be referred to as 'pracs') I had a full blown panic attack. I was so far out of my element I could barely get the words, 'I'm having a panic attack', out to my demonstrator, who looked like he might have a panic attack himself and ran to find the lab manager. I'd heard rumours about this lab manager that she was a tyrant, but actually she was very kind to me and I will be forever grateful to her for that kindness. In spite of that, I cried in 60% of first year chemistry pracs and a few of the biology ones too. My poor lab partners! Still, I got 97 for chemistry and, apart from the pracs, I loved it. Chemistry made sense in my brain; I liked the order of it. The subject was well run too and I appreciated the security of its structure.

Anxiety is part of CAPS, by the way. Aside from doctor-related anxiety (these days often talked about as medical PTSD), I almost always carried a dread feeling in the pit of my stomach. My Dad used to describe it as a flipping stomach, which is exactly what it felt like. I know it's part of CAPS because, while I still get anxiety, the flipping stomach sensation rarely happens on Kineret.

With full focus and careful time management, I completed first year with high distinctions and transferred to the Bachelor of Science (Biomed). My friend Jack did the same. Second year was a significant jump in difficulty but again I managed high distinctions, in spite of completely misunderstanding an essay instruction (i.e., and, e.g., are not the same thing) that resulted in my lowest mark for the degree of 11.5/20. Even that was a pity grade because my marker could see I had well-researched the topic and the writing was good, if misguided. The topic was experimental design. Understanding the validity of controls and what could actually be inferred from experimental work did not come naturally to me. Thanks to an excellent first year philosophy topic called 'Argument and Critical Thinking', sadly no longer offered, I could at least be aware that I was flawed with bias and, particularly with my vested interests, I would need to remain aware of this in my scientific endeavours.

The prac stress continued. Why were pracs so difficult? I'll tell you why. I still had CAPS. Things that are difficult for me include: staying upright for 4 hours straight; bright fluorescent lighting; air conditioning vents; uncomfortably high workstations with slippery, runaway chairs; unfamiliar computers; being expected to learn and immediately apply knowledge with work to be submitted during the session, without time for quiet reflection and processing. Plus the pracs were generally run in the afternoon and the end of the day is when my brain leaves me and my body says stop. I can't believe I haven't even mentioned the circadian nature of this disease. There are probably heaps of things I've forgotten to say because (a) there's a lot of it and (b) it's my normal and I forget it's not your normal. The other thing happening to me every afternoon was my abdomen swelling up like a balloon, which I hid well under bright, distracting dresses. My saving grace on prac days was my wonderful husband picking me up to drive me home, saving me the struggle of public transport. Catching a bus at the end of a prac meant a full bus and standing room only. I do not look disabled and am not elderly so there is no reasonable expectation for anyone to stand up for me. But it was excruciating.

I did some work in a genetics lab during second year. I didn't realise at the time how much bonus education I was getting because I was out of my element and full of anxiety. As is usual for me, I found it difficult to relate to the people in the lab, through no fault of theirs. They were all nice to me, and so patient. Then the most amazing thing happened. I was offered a summer placement at a lab in Brisbane that studied my gene (Fig. 5). During first year, I had travelled to the Garvan Institute of Medical Research in Sydney to attend the inaugural Australian Autoinflammatory Symposium. I'd seen that Dr Hal Hoffman from the USA was going to be presenting and, to my mind, he is the king of CAPS. If you are reading this as a young student, let me give you one piece of useful advice for your life and your career.

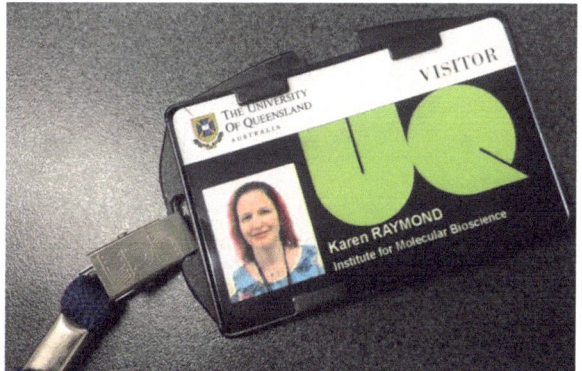

Fig. 5 My official pass to the Institute for Molecular Bioscience. That really happened

Make the effort to go and meet and talk to people in your field. Now, back to me. At the Symposium I'd not only met Dr Hoffman but also introduced myself to Associate Professor Kate Schroder, as she was then known. Her talk had fascinated me but gone largely over my head, as I had barely finished first semester of first year. I'd had to fly home the same night so I wouldn't miss my chemistry exam the next morning, which I did with a migraine for my trouble. It was worth it, fast forward 18 months and there I was doing a placement in her lab. I will say I was completely overwhelmed and enthralled by the experience, which I will never in my life forget. But I was old and sick and punching above my weight. The team of researchers there were amazing and what I learnt was that they didn't need me. Not on the bench anyway. I am going to be honest here. I am rubbish on the bench. I'm not sure if that's why I also don't like bench work but there it is.

While I was in Brisbane, Paul's Dad had a health episode that put him in hospital, which is where he was when I returned home. Sadly, he could not return home and, because I had time, I helped transition him into a nursing home. This was early 2019 and, due to a bad flu season that year, nursing homes in Adelaide began mandating flu shots. I'd never had a flu vaccine before; it just hadn't ever occurred to me.

Because of the summer experience, I entered third year with a lot more confidence, particularly where lab work was involved. I no longer cried in pracs, although

Fig. 6 Kira (left) and me. I ♥ Kira

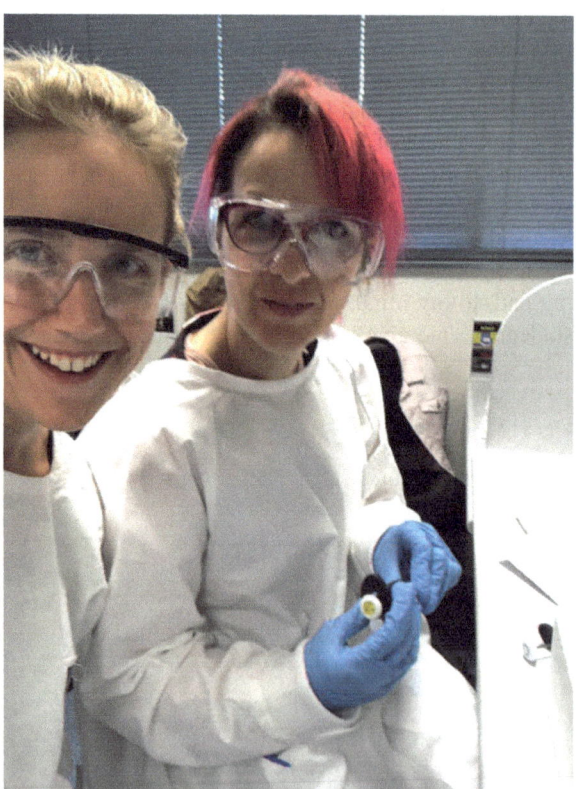

cutting the testicles out of a recently killed mouse in genetics brought me close. Thank goodness for my awesome lab partner, Kira. Instead of pracs for biochemistry, we were allowed to do placements. Kira and I got permission to do ours as a pair, which was even better (Fig. 6).

We did our experiments and were ready to present, when I came down with what I think was the flu. It felt nastier than a cold, but I didn't get a swab to check, I just stayed home. Kira was happy we got an extra week to prepare our presentation and I recovered faster than Paul, who had given the thing to me. One of the few benefits of having a hyperactive immune system, I guess.

The week after Kira and I had given our presentation, Paul and I were both over our infections and so we popped into the local pharmacy to get our flu shots, for his Dad's nursing home. No biggie. About 3 weeks after that my gut problems took a dramatic turn for the worse. I was still bleeding but now I was really jammed up, constipated. All I could get out was blood and mucus and the pain down my left side was becoming intolerable. I was part of another group project for biochemistry and during our presentation I was in so much pain I can hardly remember anything except how glad I was to be by the wall so it could hold me up. I was fully leaning on it and would have thought it odd if I'd seen someone else doing it, but I guess I was a bit of an oddball so maybe it wasn't out of character. Some post-grad students from the lab were there to critique our presentations and when I saw them a year later one of them said he had no idea I was struggling.

5   2019 Health Crisis and Publishing my Case Study

It was almost mid-semester exams and I had to work in my office while revising, as we were waiting for a new office person to start. The weekend before my first exam, the abdominal pain got so bad that I agreed to let Paul take me to hospital. After some hours, the young doctor in emergency wrote me a prescription for panadeine forte and sent me home. I went back the next day and was admitted, staying for nine nights while they unsuccessfully treated me. Not one of them had heard of CAPS and my autoinflammatory condition was not given any consideration in context of what was happening to me. I was discharged in worse shape than when I had arrived, with no pain medication. I spent two nights at home in sleepless agony, causing great distress to my husband. The first night I was hallucinating and believed the hospital had sent me home to die. My sister stepped in and demanded pain medication from the hospital. With Tramadol barely touching the pain through the second night, she contacted my gastroenterologist, who directed me to one of our private hospitals, where I could be admitted under his care.

The look on his face when he saw me in ER told me everything I needed to know. I was in terrible shape. His strategy was to completely rest my gut and put me on an elemental diet, which seemed smart. He also put me back on IV steroids and increased the azathioprine dose they'd started me on at the first hospital, which I didn't love but I complied. I was on the good pain meds (a rotation of endone, fentanyl, morphine and tapentadol) but it took weeks to get the pain under control. The crashes were horrific. After another scope, it was clear that things had gone from bad to worse and it occurred to me that I might not live through this. He said there was a drug he could give me called infliximab, but that I would have to stop taking Kineret as these drugs were contraindicated. I argued, reasoning that without Kineret my CAPS wouldn't be managed. He went away for the weekend and the doctor on duty told me sternly that if I didn't have the infliximab I would likely get cancer and/or die. I said I wanted the infliximab and could have it with the Kineret, but he wasn't having it. So I agreed to stop Kineret and they ordered the infliximab. In the meantime, I was having potassium infusions that took hours and kept the IV machine beeping all night. I was badly sleep deprived and between that, the steroids and the pain meds, I felt like I had completely lost my mind. I no longer had fine motor skills and my shakes were so pronounced that I could see the concern in the faces of my visitors. So much blood had been drawn from me that I needed a blood transfusion, which made me feel so good I started dancing on the landing outside the ward, much to the embarrassment of my visitors. Without Kineret, I had become incredibly uncomfortable and my getup was a hospital gown, a thick dressing gown, possibly Ugg boots or thick socks, I can't quite remember. I used hospital towels to wrap up my hair, not because I had washed it but because I was constantly drenched in sweat and the sweat made me too cold. My bed was under a vent that I could not control and Mum thoughtfully brought me a luxurious blanket to hide under whenever the vent came on.

The infliximab was working. I had two doses in hospital and things were getting better, but my inflammatory markers weren't coming down. I knew what the final piece of the puzzle was and I asked Paul to bring in some Kineret for me. He was nervous about it but trusted my knowledge and I reminded him that Kineret has a short half-life. If it wasn't good, it would be out of my system quickly. My kidneys have never shown signs of struggle, so I shot up Kineret and within 24 hours my inflammatory markers came down. It was 4 days before I admitted to my gastroenterologist what I had been doing. He looked at me with what I think was disappointment, but he is a pragmatic type. He said it would not be the first time a patient hadn't done as instructed and he made a note in my file. Kineret was charted for me and I no longer had to hide it. I was discharged from hospital three days later, colon intact, but with a long road to recovery ahead.

My thoughts turned back to Uni. I had been corresponding with my disability officer and some of the university staff to keep them apprised of my progress. Most of my emails contained inappropriate professions of love because the pain meds had removed my filters. The advice I'd received was, because I hadn't been able to attend my exams for genetics and biochemistry, I'd have to repeat the whole semester. It seemed harsh but there was not much I could do about it. I got an email from my second year biochemistry teacher, who had found out about my predicament and kindly reached out to check in on me. She said there was no way I would be repeating the whole semester, that I could sit the exams whenever I wanted to and I was not to hurry my recovery. Despite my *c'est la vie* attitude, this certainly reduced some stress. I don't need to be on pain meds to say how much I love her.

So, I spent time with my five cats but couldn't pick up a book to study for several months. My brain was mush; I couldn't keep a thought in my head and the shakes were still bad. It took me until November to get completely off all meds bar Kineret and infliximab, which is around the time I sat my exams. My friends had gone on to finish second semester and were graduating while I sat my first semester exams and went home again to rest and convalesce. I had my cats vaccinated and a few weeks later one of them had a metabolic crisis, requiring urgent hospitalisation. The vet thought he had developed diabetes but when insulin didn't turn things around he thought perhaps an autoimmune disease like Cushing's syndrome. We had him put down in January 2020 and it made me think back to my flu shot and the timing of that in relation to my own health crash.

I had already decided to write and publish a case study paper about my ordeal. My aim was to provide a clinical precedent, since we had resolved the issue with two contraindicated biologics that would not have happened if I wasn't me. In that paper (Raymond and Martin 2021) I did allude to the flu shot but also that I'd had what I thought was flu not long before the vaccine. Vaccines are very clever but obviously come with risks and, with my immune system being somewhat prone to going off chops, I couldn't help wondering if the flu shot or the flu (or both) had levelled up the bleeding bum issue, which had been going on for 5 years. The bleeding completely stopped while I was on both infliximab and Kineret, right up until I developed antibodies to the infliximab. [3]

In the meantime, the SARS-CoV-2 pandemic began. My Dad had started experiencing gut pain and thought he was crashing in the same way that I had done. We got him to hospital and, because of the COVID-19 restrictions, only one visitor was allowed to be with him the entire period of his admission and, because I'd accompanied him there, that was me. The emergency room doctor breezed in; he'd looked at Dad's CT scan and said some stuff about the cancer and I can't remember any of the stuff he said because he'd casually said cancer as if we knew about it. He breezed out again, leaving Dad and I blinking at each other in surprise. Dad was the first to break the shocked silence, trying to sound casual as he said, 'Everybody dies, Karen'. He didn't make it out of hospital. Turns out my Dad not only had a rare autoinflammatory disease since birth, he also had a rare cancer [4] burning away, possibly for many years, that manifested in ascites at its end stage, which is where he was at when he landed in hospital. Ascites is Greek for wine bag. In medicine, it looks like Fig. 7.

So Dad died and COVID-19 all but shut down my business. I busied myself by writing my case study paper and forced my brain back into gear for the final

---

[3] I stupidly had my 2021 flu shot too close to the infliximab infusion. We tried a different biologic, vedolizumab, which targets integrins in Peyer's patches to make the gut less permeable to immune cells, but it didn't work and I got back in remission with a different anti-TNF drug, golimumab, which lasted about a year.

[4] Dad's cancer was malignant peritoneal mesothelioma. Was he exposed to asbestos or was this yet another hyperactive mutant NLRP3 thing? Did getting him on Kineret slow down his decline or maybe speed it up?

Fig. 7 Dad's wine bag

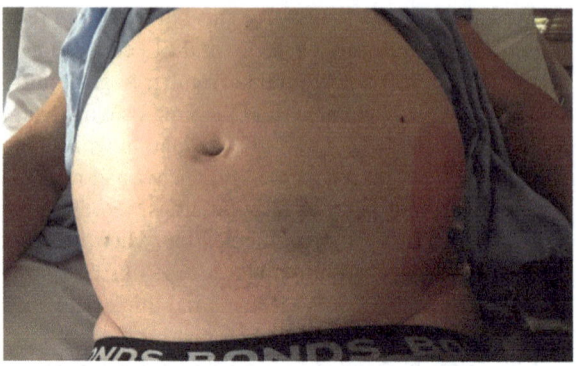

semester which, because of the pandemic, would be delivered online. I can't say I was unhappy about that, at least. Physically turning up anywhere is hard. I probably should explain that a bit more. Introverts and people with anxiety will understand it well, but the CAPS added bonus of being upright and present among others comes with the extended torture of general physical discomfort, pronounced fatigue and the toll you know it is going to take on your body later when nobody else is around. Not many things are worth that pain anymore.

The first biochemistry lecture from my favourite third year lecturer talked about hypoxia, inflammation and cancer. The official cause of death on my Dad's certificate says hypoxia, plus he had an inflammatory disease and cancer. The walls of my compartmentalisation came down and, 5 minutes in, tears were streaming down my face. Better at home in private than in a lecture theatre surrounded by students. I mean crying in pracs is one thing but in a lecture? It just wasn't done. Also, students are generally quite young and don't have the life experience to connect to much of the material and I do envy them for that.

I finished the degree, managed a perfect GPA and got the idea that I could go on and do Masters. The idea of getting a PhD appealed to me, not least because I could finally render moot the anachronistic question about whether I'm a Miss, Ms. or Mrs. I found a great lab where I could do my thing, kind of adjacent to what they were doing. Just before the pandemic, I'd attempted a placement, but struggled to cope with the demands of lab life. The next year I tried again and found I still couldn't cope with the physical requirement of being present in the lab. I still have CAPS. It's hard to be upright, under harsh lights and still so far out of my element. Add to that the lab smells and not having anyone to work with. I felt like a third testicle most of the time and had to ask myself why the hell I was putting myself through this. There is plenty of research to do but as I've said, they don't need my help on the bench. Research isn't the bottle neck when it comes to better drugs. Better drugs are coming. Awareness and education among doctors and patients is what's desperately lacking, especially here in Australia.

5.1 After Uni and Now What?

I hadn't done the degree for nothing. Most people do their study and go off to find jobs. That had never been my motivation for studying. Trying to turn up at the lab day after day had drummed it home to me that I didn't have the physical stamina needed to be consistently upright. It's hard for me to accept that I'm not able to work and it's not something I can or do explain to other people. I don't look sick. Actually, I'm a bit fabulous. I know what I'm dealing with in my daily life, so I frequently remind myself how awesome I am. The last thing I need to do is go, cap in hand, to some bureaucratic organisation asking for help. So I'm lucky that I don't have to. But I'd be lying if I didn't admit it sometimes plays in the back of my mind. What if I needed financial assistance, would I get it? I don't like being stuck on expensive medication that costs the taxpayer, even though I also pay tax to subsidise health costs for others, their kids and all the community services I don't use and make no grudges about it. It's called society and I'm a part of it even if I don't feel like it a lot of the time. So, how to contribute?

I decided my talents could be used in the area of patient education and advocacy, as this is lacking for rare diseases in general and, for CAPS in Australia, it's non-existent. I tried to step up in patient Facebook groups to help with questions being asked by patients, as my Dad had done, but that area is already well covered by the admins in the various groups [5] and, like the researchers, they don't need my help. In early 2022 I decided to start a YouTube channel [6] with the objective of demystifying the science for other CAPS patients, without them having to do the degree. The bonus would be that it would keep me motivated to stay up to date with the research. Without being connected to a lab I don't have anyone to talk to about this stuff, nobody with my fixation. So I try to remember how I felt when I was first diagnosed and didn't know what a point mutation was. Instead of making my videos perfect, I'm just making them. Everything NLRP3 and CAPS.

I also spend quite a lot of my time communicating with other CAPS patients. I've had several patients in crisis reach out to me because of my case study paper. There is frequent concern that doctors are not across the nature of an autoinflammatory disease, the quiet devastation of its low grade inflammation and the fury of its cytokine storm in a flare. In 2022 an important guidelines paper (Romano et al. 2022) was published on the management of autoinflammatory diseases and all doctors and patients need to know about it. As for me, I ended up losing my colon, a little over 8 years after the bleeding began. Post-surgery the gastroenterologist said my emergency presentation had been unusual for ulcerative colitis. Shocker. Rare diseases rarely have happy endings, we just hope for better for the next generation.

---

[5] The US-based Autoinflammatory Alliance is the go-to for autoinflammatory diseases worldwide http://www.autoinflammatory.org/. An Australian group is in its infancy under the banner of the FMF & AID Global Association http://www.fmfandaid.org with a private Facebook group called Autoinflammatory diseases AUS/NZ.

[6] http://www.youtube.com/@NLRP3.

References

Booshehri LM, Hoffman HM. CAPS and NLRP3. J Clin Immunol. 2019;39(3):277–86.

Gottschall EG. Breaking the vicious cycle. Baltimore: Kirkton Press Ltd; 1986.

Raymond KN, Martin JED. Cryopyrin-associated periodic syndrome with inflammatory bowel disease: a case study. Open Access J Gastroenterol Hepatol. 2021;5:629–31.

Romano M, Arici ZS, Piskin D, Alehashemi S, Aletaha D, Barron K, Benseler S, Berard RA, Broderick L, Dedeoglu F, et al. The 2021 EULAR/American College of Rheumatology points to consider for diagnosis, management and monitoring of the interleukin-1 mediated auto-inflammatory diseases: cryopyrin-associated periodic syndromes, tumour necrosis factor receptor-associated periodic syndrome, mevalonate kinase deficiency, and deficiency of the interleukin-1 receptor antagonist. Arthritis Rheumatol. 2022;74(7):1102–21.

To Be, or Not to Be, that Is the Question: Stuttering Into Academia

Grant Meredith

Abstract In this chapter Grant Meredith, the discipline leader of Information Technology for the Global Professional School at Federation University (Australia) outlines his journey as a person who stutters from his rural Australian upbringing through to being an Information Technology academic. This passage to academia is a reflection on an unconventional odyssey that has meandered from blue collar careers to a university education and beyond. The author discusses what it means to him to have vocal difference and how it may have influenced his research path. Along the way he questions his identity as a person who stutters and find his own "community" to engage within.

Keywords Stuttering · Stammering · Education · Academic · Pedagogy

1 An Important Preface

Before embarking on this journey of reflection and discovery, it is important to know who I, the researcher, am and how I came to be motivated to become an academic. I want to add truth to any immediate assumptions that you may have about the influences and motives for my eventual research path. This may be seen as an unconventional start to a chapter, but I believe that it is the best way to contextualise who I am and to engage you as the reader into investing the time required to continue to read on. So, I begin writing this chapter sitting alone in my home office perplexed within my own thoughts and beliefs with one broad question in my mind. How did I become an academic, who just happens to stutter? I hope to help answer this question for you throughout this narrative and present enough insight for you to form your own opinion. I will bare my life open to you all with the hope to inspire others to follow their own passions and beliefs.

G. Meredith (✉)
Global Professional School, Federation University, Ballarat, VIC, Australia
e-mail: g.meredith@federation.edu.au

© The Author(s), under exclusive license to Springer Nature Singapore Pte
Ltd. 2024
A. Stranieri et al. (eds.), *Research Partners with Lived Experience*,
https://doi.org/10.1007/978-981-97-0033-2_4

Here I sit in yet another committee meeting. "Another?", you may ask. Yes, one of the countless academic committees and working groups of which I am currently a sitting member of. Yet, after sitting in over 17 years of various meetings of all levels and purposes, I still feel a slight sense of apprehension. Apprehension, despite that this is an online meeting which has been my normality since COVID-19 changed the world and education forever. I believe it is because this is the first time that this committee has sat and that there may be some members who I have never met before, or new points of business to focus on. You may wonder whether I have a form of social anxiety or related stresses. I do not, as far as I am aware, have any such issues to manage and in fact I am known for my cool headedness amongst my colleagues. Are these feelings in fact, simply like those that we teach our students to understand in professional communication classes? I am an experienced academic, I have lectured internationally and was once an Associate Dean (Student Retention and Success). Currently I am a Discipline Lead for a new school focused on national and international partnerships. How can I have such fears, thoughts, and apprehensions, if but fleeting? I can only assume that I have these feelings because I am a person who stutters and despite all my confidence, I still at times feel a little apprehensive in new professional settings. Although I do find online meetings less stressful due to the nature of simply sitting in front on a laptop and not seeing people in person. Perhaps anxiety is felt more subconsciously than consciously? But again, are these simply natural apprehensive feelings shared by the majority in such circumstances? I believe that I am overthinking this scenario by trying to find a cause.

I am always unsure about how a person may react when first identifying that I have a very overt stutter. But to be honest, it is not at the forefront of my daily mind. Some days I do not realise that I have a stutter until something jogs my memory. I have an overt stutter which at times can show long forced speech blocks and extreme facial grimaces. Stuttering is viewed as a neurodevelopmental disorder that is complex in development with growing bodies of knowledge focusing on genetic mutations and neurological causes (Chang et al. 2019; Packman et al. 2022). In fact, I would be in a tongue-in-cheek way, a "triple threat" regarding stuttering talent as I prolong, block and repeat words, sounds, and syllables. I recognise that at times understandable reactions from peers do have a short-termed negative effect on my immediate demeanour. The notion of being an overt or covert person who stutters is debated in online stuttering communities and can be subtle in definition (Sønsterud et al. 2022). Personally, I believe there is no such binary classification of stuttering behaviours for an individual and that we moved between them fluidly due to circumstance (Meredith 2015). I am a covert overt in a sense that yes, I am openly a person who stutters. However, people do not identify me as such once they get to know me as an individual. Subconsciously, I probably simply fear negative appraisal from my fellow colleagues. Universities can be at times very judgemental to work within and assumptions may be made about talent, worth and ability to work collegially. I believe that the academics who are reading this will be able to quickly sympathise with how cut-throat and elitist academia can be. Despite these challenges, these apprehensive thoughts within me are but fleeting and I doubt that anyone would acknowledge that these little concerns even exist. On the surface I am calm and collected, measured and sometimes proudly controversial. But I ask you the reader. Is this identity just a mask that I conveniently wear at times to hide my true nature? For this chapter will be a journey of identity into an unconventional way of finding a new community and an unexpected journey into academia.

2   In the Beginning

To begin this narrative, I believe that I should share with you my upbringing and life to academia so that you can understand the factors that influenced who I was pre and post PhD. I had always been a socially outgoing and confident child who could communicate freely and jovially. Suddenly around the age of seven I became aware that I was stumbling over words and phrases when speaking at home and in class, not unlike commonly reported stuttering onset cases (Saad and Omaima 2019). Children can adapt well to changing circumstances and my peers were either not noticing or if so, not caring. Over the years throughout childhood my general speaking confidence did not drop, but from the point of self-awareness, I was fully conscious of my developing stutter, which slowly evolved over time with varying different behaviours. My family either did not notice my stumbling or they simply refused to acknowledge it. To be honest, even at this youthful age I was not sure what was happening, why it was occurring or what it was called.

Around the time of that awakening, I remember seeing an episode of the popular American historical drama television series called "*Little House on the Prairie*" and seeing a girl who stuttered on an episode called "*The Music Box*" (season 3, episode 19). I did not make the mental connection at that point that I also stuttered. I remember vividly that the episode alluded to the fact that stuttering was easily "fixed". During my growing maturity I did not identify with the portrayals of people who stuttered. I must admit though that when the 1988 diamond heist comedy was released called "*A fish called Wanda*", that Michael Palin's portrayal of stuttering Ken did resemble my own speech characteristics. Nor did I recognise any other children at my school who stuttered or know anything of the stuttering heritage within my own family. It is only of late that I realised that an uncle stuttered. I just thought of his speech as being "not the same" as others and did not bat an eyelid. He was simply an uncle who I saw a handful of times every year and was always nice to me. Yet, I knew back then that something was developing within me that made me "different" to the other local kids.

3   A Country Life

I grew up on the outskirts of Beaufort, which is a small rural farming town in Western Victoria, Australia with at that time a population of just over 3000. The town had all levels of schooling from kindergarten through to high school year 12 and attracted students from a wide rural catchment area. Throughout primary school my speech was, surprisingly, not much, if any of an issue to myself or classmates. I believe, that since I was raised in such a small country town with associated community values and because my stuttering during that period was not severely overt all the time meant that I was never really picked on because of it. It was a tightknit community in which everybody knew everybody else with a keen sense of country comradery and resilience between us all. I was picked on for things other than stuttering, including my woeful, mother-influenced, fashion sense and home-styled haircuts from my father due to the low socio-economic nature of my household. In general, my fellow students and town were fully accepting of who I was and/or were while ignoring my "different" way of speaking. The class of students who I grew up with were also a "tight unit" with most of us being together through our entire primary and secondary education years. I knew every one of the 300 plus kids at my school by name.

Reflecting on those times, I remember in upper primary school that some of my friends and I were picking on a new kid who had an obvious lisp. Which I now recognise as a clear state of bullying, and I apologise for that. Yet, then in my youth, I never really identified it as such a mean action and contradictory in nature. So, there I was, a kid with a stutter, picking on a new classmate with a lisp and with what we thought of as a slight English accent! I was a community "insider" and had the social acceptance that this new "outsider" lacked. I regret the introduction to my school that this kid received and although quickly accepted he was always given nicknames that reflected his speech impairment and accent. But I never carried such a burden on my shoulders. I do not recall meeting or recognising anyone else who had a stutter during my childhood. Later I would identify at least two other kids in lower years who did stutter. Although they stuttered, I felt no personal connection to them. As mentioned earlier, only of late have I realised that one of my uncles did have a form of stuttering. I never recognised his speech pattern as being different when I was young and would travel to Melbourne for family functions. I just thought the "umms" and "aahs" were simply how he spoke. I only recently had a revelation that his speech pattern was different to the norm. Reflecting on previous family gatherings, I never remember anyone speaking of his stuttering or having known of him being treated differently because of his speech. Nor did he ever approach me about my evolving stuttering for discussion. I guess in my family it was one of those old-fashioned unspoken issues.

My high school years, which were in the same small country town, were also filled with similar ongoing support and acceptance by teachers and fellow students like I had experienced throughout primary school. I remember doing some well received and personally satisfying presentations and debates during these hormone-driven times of adolescence. As my stuttering behaviours developed and changed, from requiring tapping a tempo out on the desk to answer a question in class through to very severe and long facially contorted blocks, I continued to be a happy and productive student. I still believe that there were some of the best years of my life without any form of adult concern. I persevered through having to read Shakespeare out aloud in English class. In fact, I was often called upon to read out aloud in class with a constant stutter due to the teacher's appreciation of my ability to read dramatic writing and to portray some emotional tone. I still laugh at having to read out a wedding invitation list in Romeo and Juliet: Act 1, scene 2 which involved a long list of names containing sounds and on almost all of which I stuttered. For example:

> Signior Martino and his wife and daughters;
> County Anselme and his beauteous sisters;
> The lady widow of Vitruvio;
> Signior Placentio and his lovely nieces;
> Mercutio and his brother Valentine (Shakespeare 2017, 1.2)

I was so vocally adept that I acted in my Year 11 drama play and often volunteered for debates, at one stage just missing out on selection for a high school radio quiz competition by a single answer. I was completely self-aware that I spoke differently to everyone else, and I was aware that everyone else knew. I was just accepted for who I was in a plain and simple country fashion. I never received any speech therapy or school-based assistance for my speech. To my surprise, I was asked during the final weeks of my final term of my final year of high school if I required any assistance to finish my completion certificate. Of course, I turned down the chance of being put onto a government funded waiting list for speech therapy at the age of 18, a month from completing high school and was slightly offended by the suggestion at that point in time. The timeline alone confused me being weeks from completion. Even with my limited knowledge of speech therapy and stuttering, I assumed that there was not much could be done for my speech within such short timeframe that may lend me an advantage in studying and completing my final examinations. Plus, *Little House on the Prairie* had taught me that supposedly stuttering could be fixed quickly and without a lot of effort.

4 Into the Real World

After completing high school, I worked in various careers, mainly those requiring strong communication skills. Most of these jobs were sales orientated and required constant and at times in-depth customer communication. I worked in male fashion sales for close to 6 months and within weeks of starting, I was competing for sales targets successfully with longstanding staff. I was not initially drawn to a career requiring a higher education degree or a large amount of further education purely because of my lack of interest at the time. I had finished high school and was unsure in which direction my life would head. I even considered the French Foreign Legion once for some adventure until I found out how much a one-way ticket to France would cost without any guarantee of acceptance. So, I worked through fashion sales, to different other retail positions and through to a range of wholesaling jobs. For almost one year I worked in retail for a florist shop and learnt so much about effective communication by having to interact with so many different customer types and differing situations requiring gifts. Working in a female dominated industry alone taught this naive young country boy a lot of communication and interpersonal skills. These situations ranged from back-room discussions to Valentine's Day rushes for gifts, and anniversaries through to funeral requirements.

I then moved into distinct roles within the wholesaling industry. The wholesaling jobs I worked within required me to visit various shops and factory sites to advertise wares and to make sure our services were meeting expectations. This career change really improved my overall communication skills and ability to have conversations with many different demographics of people at their own levels. Please keep in mind that my stuttering had been professionally rated by a speech therapist when I was in my early 20s as being quite severe as I stuttered on 33% of spoken syllables when I was rated. I was interested at that time if there were any "easy" ways to address my stuttering as I was lightly contemplating travelling overseas to work and was unsure how it would be viewed within diverse cultural situations. As a result, I found out that there was no easy fix at all for my speech and that it would require a lifelong focus on using speech management and fluency techniques in which I was not interest in investing my time within.

5 Time to Be Schooled

I decided to enrol at university as a mature-aged student while in my early 30s to instigate a career change towards information technology. Some friends of mine had just recently graduated from a Bachelor of Computing and I thought that I may as well follow their lead and improve my future career options as a result. I had also been working in my spare time doing multimedia development and had been building a portfolio both professionally and personally. The thought of moving forward with those interests seemed very appealing at the time. I entered this new adult-filled educational environment with my usual high social and speaking confidence. I remember noting on the enrolment form that I could tick a box indicating that I was "disabled" and struggled to think exactly what was meant by that. Only one thing came to mind in my case, and I thought for a moment guessing that stuttering was not a disability and I also assumed, based upon my previous school experiences, that no help was available. A somewhat ignorant and blasé view knowing what I know and have researched since (Meredith 2019; Meredith and Packman 2015). Also, without any knowledge of what advantage in schooling that I may gain from such a tick box. I did not see any real value in flagging my "disability". I thought to myself, what would they do with such information, why do they want to know that in general and would it influence my enrolment selection? Assuming that stuttering is not a disability and that there was no help available were themes that resonated strongly throughout my future PhD focus, as does the fear of discrimination based upon flagging your differences. I guess I was also a little confused about why I would check the box at all in my circumstance, the advantages of doing so or the disadvantages of not.

Throughout my three years of undergraduate study, I faired very well from a vocal point of view, and I did not have to rely on help or provision to achieve solid results. I asked questions aloud, answered questions openly and gave verbal presentations. To achieve these results, I had to focus on my classes, study hard and submit my assessment items on times. Clear and simple strategies that I teach to students even now as a lecturer. They were simple and effective study skills incorporating time management and project planning. In this adult-orientated educational world, I felt similarly treated to the way I had been treated during my primary to secondary years by my peers. No one seemed to care about how I spoke, but occasionally there was the odd social grin or chuckle at my speech. I was, however, accustomed to such responses like those I had encountered most of my life by people who did not know me or were simply not used to seeing a person stuttering. These were completely natural and understandable responses to my stuttering. We humans notice each other's human differences and react both consciously and unconsciously in response. Let's be honest with each other. There are few true saints in the world, and I can bet that all readers of this chapter have chuckled at a person who is different to the "norm" in either appearance and/or behaviour. Nor did I feel discriminated against by lecturers or marking rubrics for oral assessments.

6 Inspired Into Research

During my Bachelor years there was a turning point in my life and that was a presentation from a senior academic who told that class about Honours projects and post-graduate study. I was so impressed by his approachable nature and enthusiasm for research. He has since become a close friend, colleague, and mentor. His presentation caused me to seriously think about continuing study and to enrol in an Honours year. I believe that I would not have been an academic if I did not attend this presentation. The Honours year focused my attention on researching academic views of learning management systems and it taught me a lot about the basics of structured research. It may surprise readers that during my Honours year I gave a mid-year presentation concerning my minor thesis and received a 100% grade. This shocked me as during this presentation, by chance I was having a particularly heavy stuttering day and blocked on almost every second word. Yet the academics marking in the audience said that they could not fault my overall presentation ability and materials. The presentation was aligned to the marking guide requirements, and I had simply achieved a high score. One of characteristics of stuttering is its unpredictable nature which for some, adds anxiety towards day-to-day interactions

(Packman and Kuhn 2009). The unpredictable speech that people who stutter face are often seen as the bane of the issue. But I prefer to think of it as a notion of excitement of not knowing exactly how each speaking situation will go. It certainly is not boring for all those involved. I still teach students today regarding public presentations to focus on the message first and then the method second. Importantly though, I tell them to present with confidence and a smile.

Once, out of curiosity, I did enquire about service provision from university disability services. I am a strategist in personality. I wished to know what assistance there was for my speech if and when I needed it. To my surprise, there were little at hand and the support that was offered was based on avoiding speaking. These strategies ranged from asking to do alternative assessment items through to being the person within my student team who clicks the "next slide" button when required during a presentation. But I was not the right person to make such judgement calls due to my confidence levels? This lack of informed and client-centric service provision for students who stutter will become a future point of my academic focus.

7   Academia Here We Come

After completing my undergraduate qualifications, I began to work as a vocational education teacher teaching information technology and eventually became a university academic, experiencing life on the "other side" from being a student. But my initial foray into teaching was nervous for me not because of my speech, but because I did not have any true teaching training or qualifications. This period was one of immense learning, experimentation, and confidence building. Luckily, I had an excellent tertiary mentor who had himself taught me and initially I followed his general style. I soon developed my own practical andragogy and within my first year of teaching I was assisting to develop a new Diploma-level programme. This led to tutoring at a higher education level and an academic appointment. I remember well my first real lecture where I taught web-design to second year Bachelor of Information technology students. To add to the stress, this class was being peer-reviewed by a senior lecturer. I stuttered and blocked all through it. I must admit that I was a little concerned about feedback due to the pressure involved to perform and thought perhaps that it was the beginning and the end. The feedback I received was so encouraging and the reviewer noted that they thought that I would not be as effective a lecturer as I am without my stutter. This shocked me and as a result I wrote about the feedback for the British Stammering Association (Meredith 2009).

This experience led me to start to understand the challenges that face both students and educators alike in creating a full inclusive educational environment for all. Early in my academic career I was appointed as the first-year coordinator for the Bachelor of Information Technology students where I often found myself counselling and intervening to assist students to have a more productive academic life inside and outside the classroom. This was the passion for inclusion and support that had led to a future appointment as an Associate Dean (Student Retention and

Success) for my then Faculty. Thus began my foray into planning and beginning a PhD degree within the education discipline as opposed to pure Information Technology. As a result of my experiences as a student who stutters and as an educator. I found the focus on an educational-based PhD project to be a natural one. In turn, I eventually developed a keen passion to aid the educational inclusion of students at need and with special needs. In the future I would describe pathways to give students who stutter a strong global voice to instigate change and in turn to make them aware that true change will only occur if they speak up and inform the systems at play.

It may be of interest to the reader that the aim of my PhD began its initial life as a vastly different proposal from what it eventually evolved into. Almost as an extension of my Honours study the original broad early aim for my PhD was to form a framework of universal design rules to assist e-learning developers to create online teaching platforms and materials, and in turn, make them more accessible with disabled users in mind. Essentially, this was about designing software applications with the Visual, Auditory and Kinaesthetic (VAK) learning model and in turn, making digital learning platforms more accessible in nature. I am an information technology lecturer after all and have a passion for lecturing. I possess a heartfelt desire for making education accessible to as many people as possible and this passion resonates throughout this study. A passion for which my own university is known for and markets from. The proposed research would have then looked at human-computer interaction design, issues of usability and the broadening of accessibility for global online learning.

8   A Different Research Tact

It was early in my PhD that I developed a keen interest in technologies to support people with special needs. I needed a demographic to focus initially upon and I decided to investigate the world of stuttering because some ideas that I had for research aligned strongly with their typical characteristics. However, there was one big problem. The problem was I was not known within the stuttering community, nor was I actively engaged within. I had previously joined some Facebook stuttering support groups as I was inquisitive about general discussion trends. So, I began to engage with conversations online and I joined the Australian Speakeasy Association to understand my local stuttering communities. Soon I became a strong online voice for stuttering advocacy and often shared my own topical views and experiences. I had found a community that I fitted into of sorts. Although I still did not feel a strong personal alignment towards, but I had found a willing and eager audience. I have since presented on a range of topics at stuttering-related conferences around the world. This would prove to be a major advantage to future studies as I soon became a trusted "insider" and a global voice.

I began working with colleagues in 2011 on virtual environments within the virtual world of *Second Life*, which at the time was gaining a lot of attention from industry and research across varied disciplines. I designed and led a development team to create the world's first stuttering support centre within Second Life called the Virtual Stuttering Support Centre (VSSC). The idea of the VSSC was to give people who stutter an online and ubiquitous way of practising their coping strategies and face feared social situations within a safe environment. The VSSC also gave stuttering organisations the abilities to host online meetings, conferences, and events. Some created virtual scenarios contained "bots" that could interact with a visitor and present them with an audio narrative to practise their speech with. Bots are simply programmed representations of virtual people. Access was through the online Second Life platform and only validated members were enabled to enter the virtual building and interactive with the available functions and with each other.

The VSSC contained a range of virtual simulations and abilities including:

- A simulated shopping experience;
- Simulated job interviews;
- Simulated random conversations;
- Meeting rooms;
- A lecture theatre.

I presented the initial virtual design and premise of the VSSC to speech therapists and people who stutter at a national and an international conference. In general, most audiences were fully supportive of the development and saw it as a great step forward for online support.

Now reader, you may be thinking to yourself "wow this sounds cool and innovative!". Well, yes it was in terms of vision, technology, and functionality. The whole exercise taught me a valuable lesson for developments to come. It hammered home to me a fundamental lesson that I now teach students to strongly avoid today. Simply, if you think it's cool, then that does not mean that everyone else will think it's cool. I got so carried away with the thought of delving into innovative technologies that I forgot to ask the target users if they in fact wanted the VSSC or would use it. It was a step too far at that time for people who stutter and speech pathologists to see it as a viable option for treatment and support.

Dear readers please remember Jeff Goldblum's famous line from Jurassic Park "*...yeah, but your scientists were so preoccupied with whether or not they could that they didn't stop to think if they should*".

9 Time to Apply Oneself

After a period of reflection on the VSSC I started to think of more radical design of support for people who stutter. One idea became very prominent in mind. A simple virtual system to enable people who stutter to narratively work through commonly feared social situations like job interviews, ordering in restaurants and asking for product details in shops. To achieve this the idea of "Scenari-Aid" was born. A simple DVD system containing a range of video-recorded narrative social situations that could be worked through when the user required. This technology could work on DVD players connected to media technologies like a TV, desktop PC or laptop. A truly portable and adaptable technology. I spoke to various members of the stuttering community globally and they loved the simplicity of the concept. So, in turn, along with assistance of colleagues I applied for a small philanthropic grant and to my surprise I was granted it. It was less than what I was hoping for, but I was used to improvising and adapting to circumstance. Plus, the funding would allow me to create 1000 DVDs and distribute them to people who stutter and related organisations free of charge.

Within 6 months of gaining the funding the team and I had designed and created the DVD for publication, and it was popular attracting international stuttering programme attention. It was such a simple design and low-tech enabling it to be widely accessible. During the period of development, I had informally shown some people who stutter the design, and one came to visit me on campus. This was a major turning point in my interest and faith in the promise of the technology. Once I was visited by a potential user and she approached me with great confidence. To be honest I could not pick up any form of stuttering in her speech. She seemed very calm and at ease with meeting me and discussing her speech. She then wanted to see Scenari-Aid for herself and give me some advice on the design. I escorted her to a laboratory room, and I showed her some sample scenarios. So, what was the turning point you may ask? Well, to my surprise I observed clear physiological changes in her demeanour when she started to watch the scenarios and work through them. Her skin had turned a pale white tone, she was physically shaking and openly stuttering while attempting to work through the scenarios. EUREKA! Scenari-Aid was achieving during informal testing what I had hoped for. Its simple level of immersion, at least for this user, was replicating real-world feelings and anxieties. In turn aggravating the underlying stuttering condition. I knew that I was onto something then.

This revelation led to the creation of the applied Technologies for Empowering People for Participation in Society (TEPPS) research programme and further grant applications to continue to develop Scenari-Aid for I knew that it had to be more accessible than a DVD. This led to my universities' first crowdfunding campaign. The team and I crowdfunded for $25,000 (AU) to put Scenari-Aid online (www.scenariaid.com) and allow free accessibility along with an expanded scenario base. The campaign was launched in 2014 and after 6 weeks it reached its goal target enabling the funding to be committed to the project. This was a significant achievement as it had embraced the stuttering community and the public to have faith in the project and in turn helped to spread awareness. It has also showed the University how crowdfunding could work for attracting public funding for projects and set strategic direction for project to come.

Later in 2014, the newly developed online version of Scenari-Aid (www.scenari-aid.com) was launched to much delight and embracement of the global stuttering community and some speech pathologists. To date the website has over 4000 registered individual and organisational members globally. In 2015 I was honoured by the university by being awarded the Alumnus of the Year for "Outstanding service to the community". Despite all this short-term success, my PhD was not progressing as planned and I had accidentally side-tracked my progress detrimentally and I knew it was time to refocus and aim for completion. Yet we know that studying a PhD part-time can be a challenge for anyone, let alone an academic, due to having to fit it in with other life duties.

10   Back to the PhD

Turning back time a little it was during the early development of Scenari-Aid that my PhD project took a sudden change of focus due to a series of fortunate events. You may remember that my original PhD focus was to develop a framework for e-learning designers to develop more accessible educational platforms. While in the initial stages of the associated literature review, I reviewed a broad range of disability action plans across all Australian public universities of the time in terms of general disability service provision and including any mention of universal application design. Along the way, I observed that there was little mention at all in terms of disability or educational provision for students who stutter or who have other commonly known verbal communication disorders. I read about quite a range of provisions for students who were mobility, hearing or sight challenged, but other conditions were less focused on or overtly mentioned. Although you could read between the lines within these guides and think of strategies to assist vocally challenged students. It was perplexing why the lack of direct guidance due to the large numbers of people who may fit this characteristic. Developmental stuttering alone is estimated to directly impact 1% of the adult population globally (Brignell et al. 2020) and then if we added in the full range of speech disorders the total percentage would be quite large. This perceived absence of support became a serious refocus for my study and it genuinely interested me. I felt a serious passion rise inside me and for weeks I pondered this mentally and formed a methodological plan. After continued serious contemplation and discussion with my supervisorial team, I decided to change topics and to focus on researching the experiences of Australian university students who stutter. But why the sudden interest and passion in the plight of students who stutter, you may ask? Apart from being a person who stutters myself I identified some strategic decisions to change topics.

Perhaps being a person who stutters myself may have influenced me to subconsciously focus on "stuttering" during the initial literature review and due to my work on associated support technologies? But the choice to change topic was more of an academic decision. I certainly did not walk into candidature with noble motives in mind to become the educational saviour of people who stutter and to be prominently known for such a passion. I must be honest with you that the plight of my fellow students who stutter was not an original idea or motive at all. In a simple clinical way, my initial literature search had identified a group of individuals for whom little research and directed guidance had been conducted and formed within the frameworks of university life. Further to that, little precise university support provision was overtly mentioned for these students on the Australian university websites that

I examined. Based on these findings, and my own experiences as a student who stutters, I understood that this is a cohort of students for whom, in general, the university experience has not been an overly satisfying journey of graduated success. But having said this, being a person who stutters myself and studying fellow people who stutter has advantages. Advantages in fact that would and have assisted my quest for knowledge. These advantages have included the willingness of the studied groups of people who stutter to be more open to truly emphasise with, understand the worth of and support my proposed studies. Often, I have seen members of the stuttering community cry out for people within its own ranks to conduct research deemed as "beneficial", "authentically" lead with what Shames (2006) describes as a strong voice of "validity". There are many people who stutter who place little emphasis on modern research because they are not seeing positive changes as a result. Some are waiting impatiently for a cure, and some simply do not understand the frameworks of rigourous and ethical research designs.

Although I believe that people who do not stutter can and do research that does benefit people who stutter. I can understand some of the frustrations vented by my fellow stuttering community. Many of whom express that if you have not lived the experience of stuttering then you cannot understand its impact upon the individual. I take a different view because I believe that simply having a stutter does not make you an expert in the condition. Yes, you have the lived experiences of stuttering, but you may not have the respective discipline knowledge to understand a scientific view of the condition or may not have the resources to do so. A view for which I face ridicule and opposition myself from within my own stuttering communities and have discussed openly at related conferences. For myself my PhD study had become a deeply personal social justice study which has made, and continues to make, true tangible positive changes in terms of disability support provision for university students, including, but not only limited to, students who stutter. Yes, the findings of this study would resonate well beyond university students who stutter and will help to shape educational pathways of a diversity of students in need of provision. In simple terms I found that students who stutter in general study the degrees that they have passion for, are successful in their studies and often move into degree-aligned career paths. Underlying these glorified paths of successes though were unfulfilled grade potentials, social isolation and regrets of not making the most of their educational opportunities. For those who sought official university help for their stuttering they found that the support system was a bureaucracy driven process of service provision by well-meaning but time poor staff.

11 In Conclusion

To end this chapter, I must circle back to the question posed in the introduction "How did I become an academic, who just happens to stutter?" I think the answer is "accidentally" or perhaps it was "fate"? I had never had the goal of lecturing or academia. Yet once I had found the path, I followed it quite naturally. Upon reflection I believe that my research passion was driven at least covertly by a need to find my "community" and to make a difference for them. Even though I still do not strongly identify as a person who stutters, I do feel an attraction to that community. Well, having said that I do not wake up as a person who stutters, nor do I spend most of my daily time thinking about it. However, underneath the bravado and confidence I do stutter and rather well in my opinion. Yet, I had found my career path and interest in research initially without community. Whatever the answer truly is, I am happy that I am where I am now and doing what I am now doing.

12   Supportive Links

Australian Speak Easy Association: www.speakeasy.org.au/
  Australian Stuttering Research Centre: www.uts.edu.au/asrc
  British Stammering Association: www.stamma.org/
  International Stuttering Awareness Day: www.isad.live/home/
  Scenari-Aid: www.scenariaid.com

References

Brignell A, Krahe M, Downes M, Kefalianos E, Reilly S, Morgan AT. A systematic review of interventions for adults who stutter. J Fluen Disord. 2020;64:105766.

Chang SE, Garnett EO, Etchell A, Chow HM. Functional and neuroanatomical bases of developmental stuttering: current insights. Neuroscientist. 2019;25(6):566–82.

Meredith G. The case of the stuttering lecturer, vol. 6. London: BSA; 2009. https://stamma.org/your-voice/case-stuttering-lecturer.

Meredith G. Stuttering pride & the need for authentic media portrayal. Paper presented at the Australian Speak Easy Convention, Canberra, Australia, 2015.

Meredith G. Managed identities: how do Australian University students who stutter negotiate their studies? Doctor of Philosophy Doctoral thesis, Federation University Australia, 2019. https://researchonline.federation.edu.au/vital/access/manager/Repository/vital:14089.

Meredith G, Packman A. The experiences of university students who stutter: a quantitative and qualitative study. Procedia Soc Behav Sci. 2015;193:318–9.

Packman A, Kuhn L. Looking at stuttering through the lens of complexity. Int J Speech Lang Pathol. 2009;11(1):77–82.

Packman A, Onslow M, Lagopoulos J, Shan ZY, Lowe R, Jones M, O'Brian S, Sommer M. White matter connectivity in neonates at risk of stuttering: Preliminary data. Neurosci Lett. 2022;781:136655.

Saad MAE, Omaima MK. Childhood-onset fluency disorder (stuttering): an interruption in the flow of speaking. Psycho-Educ Res Rev. 2019;8(3):11–3.

Shakespeare W. Romeo and Juliet, act II, scene II. The Oxford Shakespeare (1914 edition). London: Oxford University Press; 2017.

Shames GH. The culture of stuttering. Paper presented at the 9th International Stuttering Awareness Day, online. 2006. https://web.mnsu.edu/comdis/isad9/papers/shames9.html.

Sønsterud H, Howells K, Ward D. Covert and overt stuttering: concepts and comparative findings. J Commun Disord. 2022;99:106246.

Living with Family Violence and The Great Escape

Elisa Zentveld

Abstract Lived experience can add an important dimension to research. Whilst acceptance of lived experience in research has not exactly taken hold yet, there is a movement towards valuing the contribution lived experience can provide, especially in some research areas. This book chapter explains how lived experience drew me, as a researcher in one discipline, to move into another research area—family violence. It is not living with family violence per se that resulted in the discipline change, but more so the systems that keep victims bound to perpetrators of family violence. I realised through my experiences that living with family violence can feel like a one-way ticket where there is no return journey; no escape route. I use my lived experience with navigating systems (namely legal systems) to contribute to family violence research. This chapter explains my three court journeys and how those outcomes and experiences led me to turn my research attention to family violence. This chapter also explains how the research gaps I uncovered could best be found through lived experience. This chapter, therefore, provides an important perspective on both the value of lived experiences with research, as well as the field of family violence (focusing on legal systems).

Keywords Family violence · Tourism · Legal system · Lived experience

1 Introduction

Sometimes researchers are drawn to a field purely through fascination. Sometimes it might be something they read that sparked a question that they wanted to solve. Some researchers are drawn to an area through personal experience of some sort. Perhaps they cared for someone with an illness or suffered from an illness and became drawn to research the field. Perhaps they suffered bullying or injustice in the

E. Zentveld (✉)
Future Regions Research Centre, Federation University Australia, Mt. Helen, VIC, Australia
e-mail: e.zentveld@federation.edu.au

© The Author(s), under exclusive license to Springer Nature Singapore Pte Ltd. 2024
A. Stranieri et al. (eds.), *Research Partners with Lived Experience*,
https://doi.org/10.1007/978-981-97-0033-2_5

workplace and became drawn to that field. In my case, as an existing researcher with almost two decades of research experience in tourism, I moved into a new discipline; that of family violence. I made that change because of lived experience and the gaps and problems I found in the systems through journeying through them.

This chapter outlines how I journeyed to use my lived experience to change from the discipline I had researched for almost 20 years, to that of family violence. In saying my lived experience, it was not so much living with family violence per se, but trying to untangle myself and my children from 'the perpetrator's web' as I call it (discussed later in this chapter). I discovered how systems, mainly legal systems, can trap victims of family violence. The pro-contact culture binds victims and victim children to the perpetrator. The process is discretionary and complex, and too many victims of family violence end up with what they consider to be harmful court orders resulting in them feeling regret for separating.

I spent the best part of three years journeying through three separate court processes to untangle myself and my children, and try to help them heal from the trauma and damage done to them caused by living with family violence. I read many cases alongside legislation to try to strategise how to untangle myself and my children, and my outcomes were so much better than so very many victims of family violence. I thought to myself—all this learning must have a purpose. The purpose surely must be bigger than just me and my children. And so, I began my journey of 'starting again' in a new discipline area, with an aim to use my experiences and learning to make a difference. This chapter tells that story.

2   Lived Experience in Research

Lived experience can be described as 'personal knowledge about the world gained through direct, first-hand involvements in everyday events rather than through representations constructed by other people' (IGI Global 2023). There has been a recent movement towards respecting the important role that lived experience can add to research. Of course, lived experience is already highly valued in creative areas. Many song lyrics are based on experiences by the songwriter. Many novels, including fiction, stem from experience. For example, whilst *Bleak House* (Dickens 1993) is fiction, the plot stemmed from Charles Dicken's experiences as a court reporter in London, where he observed drawn-out court cases. Furthermore, the 2017 French drama/thriller film *Custody* was enrichened by the research efforts of the Director, Xavier Legrand, who sat in family violence court cases as an observer to better understand what happens to inform his writing the film script.

Thus, lived experience and personal observation can be highly regarded in creative works. However, lived experience has not yet reached that level of respect in the research world, where some might believe research involves being entirely detached from the subject matter. Accordingly, the integration of lived experience into traditional scientific data analysis has not exactly taken hold yet, although there has been some slow movement towards recognising how lived experience can be an important aspect of research.

Our traditional understanding of research is that 'systematic reviews and meta-analyses are considered the highest levels of scientific evidence' (Beames et al. 2021, p. 1). Individuals who have lived experience are not usually involved in the underlying method (Beames et al. 2021). This can result in some gaps or deficiencies.

For example, let's imagine we wanted to do a study on what it is like to walk on the moon. We could look at images taken, draw on analysis, and use scientific tools to draw hypotheses for our research. We could allow our research to draw conclusions. Now imagine we considered lived experience. Out of the 24 people who have been to the moon, ten are still alive as of the time of writing this book chapter. Imagine if one of those people wrote the research report—developing the narrative as they deemed appropriate and outlining what has been learned and what is needed. If one of those ten living astronauts presented a study about being on the moon, I think it is fair to say that this might be valuable compared with no lived experience.

It's an extreme example, but it highlights how advantageous lived experience might be in some situations. I would also argue that lived experience in some research areas may be especially critical. For example, imagine being a researcher developing a study to investigate the process of parenting a child who wants to change gender. The researcher could read existing literature on what conceptual framework to use, what questions have been asked in the past, what methods have been previously employed, and what research gaps there are in the field. Contrasting that, imagine that the researcher has lived experience. It is reasonable that the research gaps they identify are ones that only someone with lived experience may realise. Some research questions might only be thought of through lived experience. Another such example is family violence, and hopefully, by the end of this chapter, readers will understand why I say that.

3   Family Violence Research

The research that has taken place into family violence is diverse and sits across various disciplines. Whilst family violence is not exclusively against a woman from a man, women are ten times more likely to be the victim rather than the perpetrator of family violence, and the abuse against women by men is more lethal (Spearman et al. 2022). There is also a gendered difference in understanding abuse, with abusive men minimising their violence and victim-blaming (Stark and Hester 2019).

There is a significant volume of literature on family violence. A simple Google Scholar search for 'family violence' produced 3,930,000 results at the time of writing this book chapter. A search for 'domestic violence' at the same time yielded 2,910,000 results. Drilling down into the post-separation aspect of family violence in Australia yielded 5390 results of which about half of those results had been since 2015.

As is evident, the results outline the great amount of work that has been undertaken in the field of family violence. It is probably important at this point to mention that I specifically use the term 'family violence'. This is for several reasons, but most particularly, because my research has focused on the legal systems relating to family violence and the Family Law Act recognises 'family violence'. There are some differences across various legislation, but in simple terms, family violence is about the relationship (i.e., family) and not the setting (i.e., it does not have to occur in a domestic setting). By contrast, domestic violence is about the setting (i.e., in the home) rather than the relationship. An example of domestic violence is two unrelated flatmates. Family violence does not need to occur between people who share a home. In fact, much of the family violence that occurs is after separation.

There is a common misconception that if someone is living with family violence, then all they need to do is leave. If only it was that simple. Leaving is not at all simple for many reasons, and 'separating from an abusive parent is often a difficult decision for women' (Broughton and Ford-Gilboe 2016, p. 2469). Much focus is on the process towards leaving an abusive relationship (Broughton and Ford-Gilboe 2016; Spearman et al. 2022) and less is known about 'how *families* work through this transition and the implications for the health and well-being of the family over time' (Broughton and Ford-Gilboe 2016, p. 2469). Leaving a situation of family violence is extremely complex, especially once there are children between the couple. Once children are involved, a key aspect will be the legal systems that determine the parenting matters. Yet, relatively little is known about the post-separation challenges for victims of family violence.

Some people may feel that separation from a perpetrator of family violence is synonymous with freedom. These people who have left a situation of family violence are often referred to as 'survivors' or 'victim-survivors'. The word survivor might present an illusion that the trouble is in the past, but this is far from reality for many victims. Various studies have found that 'survivors, especially those with pain, often suffer from depression and other psychiatric disorders such as posttraumatic stress disorder' (Cerulli et al. 2012, p. 773). Thus, the term 'survivor' or even 'victim-survivor' can seem a little ill-placed as some people do not relate to those terms and feel that the internal and external scars are too significant to feel like a survivor (Zentveld 2023).

In many cases, separation creates a different type of trauma where 'the abuser was relentless by retraumatising the victim repeatedly through shared parenting, prolonged court cases, etc.' (Cerulli et al. 2012, p. 773). In a study undertaken by Broughton and Ford-Gilboe (2016), the majority of women who had separated from their abusive partner continued to experience family violence despite having separated on average 2.5 years prior. In fact, some women feel that the abuse will never be over: 'when we went through everything at court, I thought it would be over. When he was sentenced, I thought it would be over. It just never is' (Cerulli et al. 2012, p. 773). Many separated women find that abuse continues after separation, and they often turn to the family court for assistance to keep their children safe, although often 'family court did not respond in ways they believed protected their children' (Zeoli et al. 2013, p. 547).

Sadly, the perpetrator remains present in the lives of victims of family violence through court-mandated child contact agreements and also harassment which will often continue. Furthermore, the trauma and emotional pain can continue for generations (Thiara and Humphreys 2017).

The pain for children living with family violence is not well understood, but it is gradually being recognised that children are impacted by family violence even if they are not a direct target of that abuse. The notion of living in a household in which the child hears and sees their mother being attacked and living with fear and unpredictability has negative impacts on the development of the child and their mental health and well-being (Mullender et al. 2002). Children who grow up living with family violence have more emotional, cognitive, behavioural, and social problems than those children who do not grow up living with family violence (Stiller et al. 2022). Witnessing family violence also contributes to children's acceptability of family violence where 'significant correlations were found between the child's belief in male power and the frequency of physical abuse and psychological abuse reported as experienced by the mother' (Graham-Bermann and Brescoll 2000, p. 607).

Witnessing family violence in the home can greatly impact a child and result in detrimental impacts on a child's attitudes, quality of life, and behaviour (Stiller et al. 2022). Problematically, court systems are often seen to fail victims of family violence whereby victims who separate from an abuser may actually regret leaving because they find they are left with harmful court orders that make life worse for them and their children (Kivela 2020). The legal systems across the globe do not appear to be adequately versed in the significant impact that family violence has on families even after separation. Research has shown that children can have nightmares, angry outbursts, poor self-esteem, and difficulty sleeping and that traumatic memories plague children long after separation (Humphreys et al. 2019). Despite violent behaviour resulting in the completion of Men's Behaviour Change Programmes (which are often court-mandated), abuse continues and women report 'problematic fathering' as well as 'very high levels of child abuse and poor attitudes to both women and children' before as well as after separating (Humphreys et al. 2019, p. 321). The family court processes, with their pro-contact mentality regardless of family violence, are often not conducive to supporting victims and children, resulting in ongoing family violence.

4   My Lived Experience

In many ways, my story begins in September 2017. By that time, I had been an academic for 12 years and living with family violence for much of my marriage (April 2001). I say much of my marriage because, like most people who find themselves in an abusive relationship, it didn't start that way. The person I married isn't who emerged over time. Looking back, there were some signs before I got married, but those small signs are only clear to me with the benefit of what I now know about family violence.

A year after being married, my then-husband stopped working and it was solely my task to earn the income. My oldest child (a male) was born in February 2003, and the next child (a female) was born the next year in November 2004. Less than 6 months after giving birth to my daughter, I discovered I was pregnant with identical twins. My then-husband did not talk to me for three days saying I was selfish for wanting to keep the babies as we wouldn't have enough money to give so many children a good life. Things really soured after that time. Without going into the details, I will summarise it by saying that there was control and abuse as well as physical episodes directed both at me and the children. There were many times I was choked. On one occasion my eldest son (who was 10 at the time) called 000 (the emergency line in Australia) after my then-husband hit me in the head causing a perforated eardrum, black eye, and cut eyebrow.

Like many victims of family violence, I was trapped in what I call the 'Perpetrator's Web' (Fig. 1). As can be seen in Fig. 1, the outside of the 'web' shows attributes that could readily bring a potential victim to the 'web'. The person can be attentive, thoughtful, loving and kind. The person is attracted to the perpetrator in some ways similar to a spider's web, where the spider can lure prey, literally. A spider's web will trap the prey once the prey is within the web, but that prey is first attracted (through electric attraction) (Garber 2013). Similarly, prey (i.e., a victim) will be lured to the perpetrator. The initial displayed qualities of the perpetrator attracted the victim and as they enter the web, a cycle begins where their less attractive attributes are revealed such as being possessive, controlling, and angry. But then they are sorry and there are gifts to demonstrate their remorse. The victim feels that the perpetrator has been misunderstood and has suffered misfortune and they often try to help that person. The victim is lured further into the centre of the web. It is at this point, the centre, where a child or children are produced between the couple which connects the victim to the perpetrator for life. The key point I want to highlight is that the person who is revealed to be a perpetrator of family violence later in the relationship, is not revealed to be such a person at the beginning when the victim meets the perpetrator or starts to date them. It is a trap, in much the same way as a spider's web is.

Once I realised I was trapped in the 'web', I had to try to work out how to escape. It was through that mental process that I realised how the 'system' (i.e., society and the family legal system) makes it difficult for victims to leave an abusive relationship. I drew on my research skills to work out how to escape family violence. When to leave; how to leave. I spent many years planning 'the great escape' and once I finally left the relationship, I then had to spend much of the next three years dealing with three separate court cases to untangle myself. Much of what I learned and observed from the 'system' came through the experiences of my children and as such the particular direction I went in as a researcher was lived with and through my children. The experiences of my daughter are captured through these words penned by her:

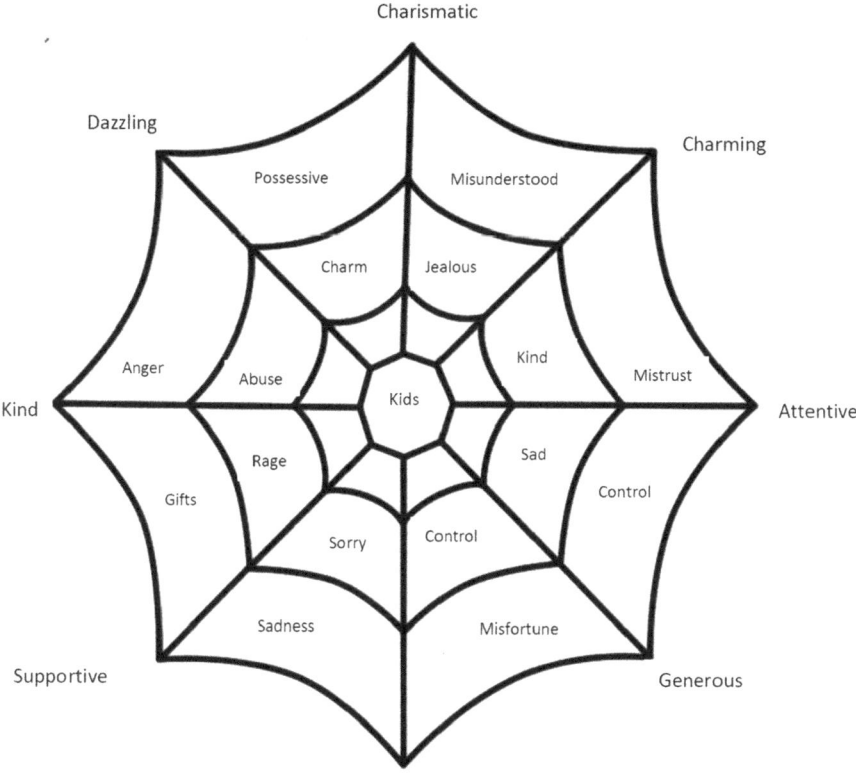

The Garden of Eden

Fig. 1 The Perpetrator's web (Adapted from Zentveld 2023, p. 57)

My childhood was a collapsed sandcastle,
    A weak foundation and broken smiles.
    Each time it was re-built,
    The tidal wave of my father's abuse
    Knocked it over again and again.
    Trampled, the sand grains turned to dust,
    Slipped through my tiny fingers,
    My childhood I lost.

I spent years with different therapists discussing my feelings, but never felt understood. They were trying to treat just my symptoms, because I never realised my symptoms had a root cause.

When I realised I had spent so many years neglecting my past, I realised my childhood trauma was the root cause of it all. After my realisation, I dedicated my spare time to better understanding myself. I would research impacts of child abuse in teenagers, and I realised how many symptoms were prevalent in my life. Low self-esteem, low self-worth, distrust, depression, anxiety, suicidal ideation, nightmares, disordered eating, as well as toxic friendships and relationships.

Whilst treating the symptoms (anxiety, low self-esteem) is necessary, I had to better understand myself first to be able to heal. For me at least, I didn't understand why I felt all these things, and once I realised that it was because my brain was developed whilst walking on eggshells, I realised that everything I felt was completely normal for any other person in my shoes, and so I accepted myself and began to work on myself.

Unfortunately, children who experience abuse often grow up with a warped view of love and life. This leads to toxic relationship patterns continuing into their teenage years and adulthood. As a child, if you witnessed fighting, screaming, anger, distrust, and all-around negativity between your parents, that becomes normal and ingrained into your mind.

My experiences caused extremely low confidence, anxiety, low self-esteem and low self-worth. This manifested into my 14-year-old self-being stuck in a toxic friendship for many years as I was never able to speak up for myself.

Researching childhood trauma opened my eyes and made me realise what I was doing, and that these present toxic situations were in fact not normal. I went to a specialised therapist who helped me unpack some of these past traumas and the way they manifested into the present, paired with my own research, helped me to understand myself on a much deeper level, and gave me the knowledge needed to heal and grow.

How do I forgive someone who took so much,
　　With no remorse or sorrow?
　　To forgive, but never to forget.
　　Unforgettable, he left his mark.
　　Bruises that went far beneath my skin.
　　Tore me down, yet my job to repair.
　　I could never understand.
　　How that could be fair.

The final piece from my daughter is so critical—'tore me down, yet my job to repair'. I have read and observed court cases relating to family violence, where the perpetrator might be required to pay for the damages to the house. I have often wondered—who repairs the brain? For example, one case involved a perpetrator damaging the front door where his ex-wife and two daughters resided. He threatened to set fire to the house if they did not let him in. I cannot imagine what terror they felt, and I wonder—who pays for the cost of the therapy caused by that perpetrator? He was court-ordered to pay for the damaged door. But he also caused the fear, and who pays for the therapy? Sadly, the victim.

As mentioned earlier, I spent virtually three years in three separate court cases trying to untangle myself from the situation. The first case was parenting/financial agreements; the second case was an Intervention Order; the third case was changing the children's surnames.

The last one was a recommendation from a child psychologist treating my daughter. My daughter was suffering from flashbacks of traumatic episodes in her childhood whenever she saw or wrote her birth surname. The psychologist recommended that I formally change the name.

All three court cases, but especially the third case, opened my eyes to the horror of family court. Many different people have told me shocking stories about the harmful court orders they were left with. Many have told me about the terrible treatment they received in court. It is still only when I experienced it myself that I understood how bad it can be.

The experiences in court resulted in my decision to use my lived experience to frame my research. Importantly, I used my lived experience to change my research where I was (and at the time of writing this, still am) listed number one in the world for my field of research. I have now, in a sense, 'started from scratch' in a new field. To understand why, I need to explain a little about my court cases. My decision to research into the area of family violence came not from living with it, but from dealing with the legal system to separate from family violence.

Court Matter Number One   In Australia, there is a Family Law Act 1975, where the default position is for separated parents to have 'equal shared parental responsibilities'. This means that separated parents must discuss and agree on the major issues for their child/ren. Things such as: religion, health, education, and name— these are the types of major things that the separated parents must discuss and decide upon. Regardless of who has the child for what amount of time, or even no time at all, the default provision is for 'equal shared parental responsibilities'. There are similar clauses in other countries but called other things. In Australia, in the Family Law Act 1975, equal shared parental responsibilities can be rebutted if there has been family violence. However, there is a legal preference to apply 'equal shared parental responsibilities' over 'sole parental responsibilities' (where only one parent makes all the major long-term decisions for the child/ren). Where parents do not go through a court process, the default of equal shared parental responsibilities applies. For those matters that go to court for decisions, 'It is extremely rare for the Court to award sole parental responsibility and operates under the presumption that equal shared parental responsibility will be best for the child' (Reardon 2021).

Perpetrators of family violence are abusive and controlling individuals. The notion of giving such individuals the power to make decisions for a child can be incredibly unsuitable. Requests for certain healthcare needs, education changes, religious matters, or other major long-term matters for the child might be denied by the perpetrator parent; they may simply not respond.

Whilst equal shared parental responsibilities may not be inappropriate in all cases of family violence, it is inappropriate in some cases. Based on the type of person I was separating from, I was of the opinion that giving him power to make decisions about the welfare of the children was not going to be in their best interests. I refused to agree to 'equal shared parental responsibilities'. I made it clear that I would negotiate on finances, but not on that point. I spent my evenings for many months reading the Family Law Act, blogs, media, and case law. I was intent on finding a mechanism to achieve 'sole parental responsibilities'.

Eventually, after almost 12 months to the day, the parental and financial matters were finalised and I had what very few parents in Australia have—sole parental responsibilities. I figured that all that reading, interpreting, strategising, and planning could not have been just to benefit me and my children. There simply had to be a bigger purpose.

Court Matter Number Two   There were two other matters in court I dealt with as part of my journey to untangle myself from family violence. One of those was getting an Intervention Order. To reduce my legal costs, I managed this process myself. My ex-husband lawyered up and in court the lawyer asked for 'further and better particulars'. I had no idea what that was and when I tried to find out at the Court reception area, I was told to ask my lawyer, which I didn't have and didn't want to have to get to save costs.

A member of staff from a family violence organisation told me this is a common tactic whereby a request is made for 'further and better particulars', which requires the person coming back to court and taking another day off work and arranging childcare another time as well as getting a lawyer. The simple way to escape this difficult situation is to drop the application. I was informed that this is the purpose of the tactic.

When I got home, I googled 'further and better particulars' and discovered that it was essentially just a report. I was so relieved as writing a report was not at all difficult. Since I was informed that the request is a tactic to try to get the matter dropped, I felt determined to continue. I put together my list of allegations and evidence and decided that if they wanted 'further and better particulars', they sure were going to get that. The document I put together was around 40 pages long. For my amusement, I had the document thermal bound. I decided to be a bit of a nuisance and make it a bit annoying for the lawyer to have to photocopy and send it to their client. I figured I may as well play some tactics back. The outcome was for a five-year Intervention Order placed against my ex-husband where he couldn't contact my parents, the children (directly), or go near our home or the children's schools. It meant he could not attend parent-teacher interviews at the school or access their school records. My learning from that was about tactics and processes and I shared this in detail in my book (Zentveld 2023).

Court Matter Number Three   The third court journey I had, which was easily the worst in terms of experience, was to change the surnames of the children. As I mentioned earlier in this book chapter, my lived experience included the impacts on my children. My daughter struggled with her birth surname and kept asking to have it changed. She refused to write her surname on school test papers, and for social media, she used her middle name as her surname. She would have flashbacks of violent episodes from her past when she saw or wrote her surname. I sent her to a child psychologist to assist her in accepting her birth surname and viewing it differently. Instead, the child psychologist told me it would be helpful to change the surname as it would likely help reduce flashbacks and empower my daughter.

That advice then pushed me into a pathway of trying to learn how to go about changing the surnames of children. The difficulty for me was compounded by the fact that two of my children were born in one Australian state (Queensland), the other two children were born in a different Australian state (New South Wales), and we lived in a different state to those two states (Victoria). Each state has its own legislation (Births, Deaths, Marriages). As far as I could tell from the reading of the legislation, the state body for changing names in Victoria would have no jurisdiction over other states.

I thought that the best chance might be at a national level—the Family Court of Australia. However, there isn't really a process for name changes in the Family Law

Act. I won't go through all the details of the journey through this matter in this book chapter, as it was a long and complex process; but interested readers can locate the journey in my book (Zentveld 2023).

This court journey really cemented my feelings about the injustice of the 'justice' system. In short, because I had already been awarded 'sole parental responsibilities' it seemed entirely reasonable that I solely apply to the court for orders to change the children's names. A previous court process had already bestowed all powers to me relating to making decisions for the major issues relating to the children (religion, health, education, name). However, the Judge wanted to invite the father to comment and this was a bit like poking a grizzly bear.

I had to locate the father in order to serve him, which was a process in itself. When I managed to make contact with him, I had to ask for an address to serve papers. He gave me a false address (which belonged to a family member of his). Respondents who wish to lodge a response to contribute to the court matter must serve and file papers at least seven days before the scheduled hearing. A few hours before the hearing, I was served lengthy response papers via email but I did not have time to read the papers nor did I make too much of them given their lodgement was well outside the timelines.

The Hearing proceeded, and the orders were granted to change the children's names. Numerous weeks later, I received a letter from the lawyer representing my ex-husband threatening various things if I did not agree to set aside the orders. It was all a bit of a nonsense given by that time the new birth certificates had arrived for two of the children with identification transitioned, and the other two birth certificates were on their way.

However, an appeal was made, which was entertained by the Judge. That began a dreadful process where the Judge seemed to be seduced by the tearful story from the father and she made orders that over-rode the previous ones (which was a matter unrelated to the name-change case). This was utterly extraordinary because the matter was a name-change application and the papers related solely to the change of names. Yet, a completely different item was ordered, not in any of the papers, which was forced weekly communication. Nothing about 'in accordance with the children's wishes' was attached to the new order. So, I was court-ordered to force four teenagers, who were still dealing with their recovery from abuse, to speak to a father they did not want to speak to. It is hard enough to get a teenager to clean their bedroom. How does someone force someone to speak to a person against their wishes? And if they refuse? Then I am breaching court orders. This was extremely concerning and irregular.

The father was in his element. He took delight in demanding to me that he wanted four weekly one-on-one calls and that a group call was not at all adequate. My daughter took the news very hard. She refused to eat and said she wanted to change her name to be free and now she had been connected back to her abuser. She then overdosed on painkillers and ended up in hospital. I hold the judicial system entirely to blame for this.

I ended up conjuring up a strategy for how to undo the new court orders. The details of this can be read in the Overture of Zentveld (2023). There was to be another hearing four weeks later to check I had abided by the new forced communication order. This presented an opportunity to turn around the situation and so I submitted papers, affidavits, evidence; and I requested the new court order be revoked. The hearing lasted only a few minutes and the orders that were made against the children's wishes vanished.

I learned a lot from journeying through the three court processes. No amount of reading or research on its own could have possibly opened my eyes to the under-belly of the problem with family violence adequately. Living with family violence, seeing its impact on my children, and then journeying through the horror of court was a learning that cannot be matched by being a detached armchair critic.

There is much about being in court that is frightening—the outcomes are never certain and the processes are unfamiliar. These can be difficult steps. The impact of court only reinforced itself to me quite recently whilst seated in a courtroom (I now do family violence court observation work as part of my research). There were delays for the first two cases and I sat for half an hour before anything started. Whilst I sat there in an almost empty courtroom, my mind went back to 2013. I was in court for the police-issued intervention order (that is a different matter to the one I write of in this book chapter). A policewoman sat beside me and said 'are you sure you want to take him back because you look really frightened'. When the case was over, I walked to where my car was parked and my then-husband walked with me, which is not at all what I wanted. He tried to be affectionate and I felt like I wanted to be teleported away. I felt nauseous. I felt miserable. That was back in 2013; and yet there I sat, in the courtroom, in 2023, merely waiting for the cases to start and I was there only as an observer, seeing myself from the past. It was as though I was watching a movie and I could see myself as the key actor in it, but it was 10 years prior. I have done court observation work before and never had this occur. I mentioned it to a person the next day and they asked whether I was comfortable going again. In my view, the flashback could only have happened because there was still some trauma to release. Perhaps there is more buried to be released as more time passes.

5   Discussion and Conclusion

As outlined in this book chapter, my lived experience journeying through court resulted in me moving across into a new discipline area. Legal research tends to be doctrinal research. It concerns the legal principle that evolves from court processes through the guiding legislation. Doctrinal research is not concerned with how people feel and whether the processes work effectively. The name-change case of mine created new case law and is published in AustLII. But it is a façade because only the first hearing where the name-change orders were made were published. The published case ends where it should have ended in real life. What happened afterwards is hidden from the world and therefore cannot possibly be found through doctrinal research.

It is my belief that family violence continues to be a problem in part because of the legal system which promotes forced contact with perpetrators of family violence. Despite their behaviour, they are granted time, often significant time, with their children. Most significantly, they are almost always entitled to co-make decisions regarding major long-term matters (e.g., health, education, religion, and name) about the child.

Some people stay living with family violence because they consider it better than risking being the recipient of harmful court orders. So, children are exposed to further family violence either through a delayed separation or through court-mandated time with a perpetrator of family violence after separation.

These things may then manifest into problematic behaviour in children as well as the ongoing cycle of patriarchy. It is alarming that:

> the amount of physical violence and emotional abuse reported to be experienced by the mother was significantly related to how much children believed in the inherent superiority and privilege of men in the family and also to how much children believed that violence was an acceptable and even necessary part of family interactions. These relationships suggest that children's cognitive belief systems, in this case around gender and family violence, may be affected by witnessing the abuse of their mothers (Graham-Bermann and Brescoll 2000, p. 609).

Thus, systems that allow more exposure to family violence are at least partially accountable for the continuation of family violence in our society. These processes highlight another layer in the difficulty of trying to separate from a perpetrator of family violence and that it is most certainly not a case of 'just leaving'. The process can be thought of as 'the great escape' (Zentveld 2023) and the equivalent of trying to climb Mount Everest.

Court in itself is stressful, and the waiting periods and imprecise nature of costings can greatly add to the unpleasant nature of proceedings. After court filings, it might be one or two months before the first hearing or in some cases much longer. The number of hearings and whether there are adjournments is unknown at the outset. Family law court proceedings may take one or two years, or even more, to resolve. Of course, family law is not the only area in which court cases may be protracted and filled with unpleasantness. Many other domains result similarly, and anyone who has read *Bleak House* (Dickens 1993), would be forgiven for wanting to avoid having anything to do with a court case. Dickens, who was a court reporter in London, also used lived experience for his work. He used his life experience from observation of court cases to develop the plot for 'Bleak House'. The novel, which centres around a complicated probate court case spanning for generations sets the scene aptly in its first chapter with 'Jarndyce and Jarndyce drones on. This scarecrow of a suit has, over the course of time, become so complicated, that no man alive knows what it means' (Dickens 1993, p. 5). The plot reveals characters connected to the case who tend to suffer a tragic fate from becoming consumed by the lust for possible wealth and the pursuit of greed despite the hurt it brings to others. The famous novel reveals lawyers with characters that nobody would want to be on the wrong side of. Whilst a fictional case, lived experience as a court reporter developed the plot. The depiction of the loss of oneself through an endless court case, even in a fictional setting, makes a powerful impression on anyone having to journey through court.

As mentioned in this book chapter, I spent considerable time researching, learning, and mapping out my great escape from the Perpetrator's Web, and journeying through three separate court cases. I figured that all that learning had to be for a bigger purpose than just me and my four children. And as such, I transitioned and 'started again' in a new research area in the hope that my experiences may serve a bigger purpose. I discovered issues that could only be discovered by riding through the court journeys in the 'driver's seat.' I hope that my lived experience through my research will help result in raising awareness about the problems with family violence, and that in time we will see safer court orders that are truly in the best interests of the child.

References

Beames JR, Kikas K, O'Gradey-Lee M, et al. A new normal: integrating lived experience into scientific data syntheses. Front Psych. 2021;12:10–3. https://doi.org/10.3389/fpsyt.2021.763005.

Broughton S, Ford-Gilboe M. Predicting family health and well-being after separation from an abusive partner: role of coercive control, mother's depression and social support. J Clin Nurs. 2016;26:2468–81.

Cerulli C, Poleshuck E, Raimondi C, et al. "What fresh hell is this?" Victims of intimate partner violence describe their experiences of abuse, pain, and depression. J Fam Violence. 2012;27:773–81. https://doi.org/10.1007/s10896-012-9469-6.

Dickens C. Bleak house. Belmont: Wordsworth; 1993.

Garber M. Confirmed: Spiders are even more terrifying than previously thought. The Atlantic. 2013. https://www.theatlantic.com/technology/archive/2013/07/confirmed-spiders-are-even-more-terrifying-than-previously-thought/277544/.

Graham-Bermann SA, Brescoll V. Gender, power, and violence: assessing the family stereotypes of the children of batterers. J Fam Psychol. 2000;14:600–12. https://doi.org/10.1037/0893-3200.14.4.600.

Humphreys C, Diemer K, Bornemisza A, et al. More present than absent: men who use domestic violence and their fathering. Child Fam Soc Work. 2019;24:321–9. https://doi.org/10.1111/cfs.12617.

IGI Global. What is lived experience. 2023. https://www.igi-global.com/dictionary/lived-experience/17273.

Kivela B. "The harm report": assessing risk of harm to children and parents in private law cases. Rayden Solicitors. 2020. https://raydensolicitors.co.uk/blog/the-harm-report-assessing-risk-of-harm-to-children-and-parents-in-private-law-cases/.

Mullender A, Hague G, Imam I, et al. Children's perspectives on domestic violence. London: Sage; 2002.

Reardon T. An expert guide to sole parental responsibility in Australia. Unified Lawyers. 2021. https://www.unifiedlawyers.com.au/blog/sole-parental-responsibility-guide/.

Spearman KJ, Hardesty JL, Campbell J. Post-separation abuse: a concept analysis. J Adv Nurs. 2022;May:1–22. https://doi.org/10.1111/jan.15310.

Stark E, Hester M. Coercive control: update and review. Violence Against Women. 2019;25:81–104. https://doi.org/10.1177/1077801218816191.

Stiller A, Neubert C, Krieg Y. Witnessing intimate partner violence as a child and associated consequences. J Interpers Violence. 2022;37:NP20898–927.

Thiara RK, Humphreys C. Absent presence: the ongoing impact of men's violence on the mother–child relationship. Child Fam Soc Work. 2017;22:137–45. https://doi.org/10.1111/cfs.12210.

Zentveld E. Control, abuse, bullying, and family violence in tourism industries. Bristol: Channel View Publications; 2023.

Zeoli AM, Rivera EA, Sullivan CM, et al. Post-separation abuse of women and their children: boundary-setting and family court utilization among victimized mothers. J Fam Violence. 2013;28:547–60. https://doi.org/10.1007/s10896-013-9528-7.

My Journey: From Patient to Researcher with Lived Experience

Truus Teunissen and Tineke Abma

Abstract As a person with multiple chronic illnesses, I, Truus Teunissen, have had to deal with the problems in all aspects of my life: at home, at work, social, and societal. Although I now see myself as a citizen living life to the fullest, it took a long time, and I still struggle, to free myself from the feeling of "being the disease." After getting involved in several patient organizations and committees, I saw that there was still much to do about meaningful and structural patient involvement in research, policy, and care practice. My drive is about caring for other people with illnesses through action research. As a PhD candidate and later as scientific researcher, I developed together with other patients a set of criteria and values. This is used in order to discuss patient perspectives in committees or platforms and for appraisal or evaluation of project proposals in health research and in health care from a patient perspective, by patients (representatives). This set of criteria and values is still in use after 12 years throughout The Netherlands. My family, friends, and co-researchers joined me on my journey to become a researcher with lived experiences. In the current main societal discourse, there are many issues to fight for when it comes to meaningful patient involvement, to living a full life despite health problems, to inclusion and justice. I still work as a guest scientific researcher, combining scientific knowledge and experiential knowledge, since investigating and understanding these issues is of paramount importance for achieving progress.

Keywords Illness · Meaningful life · Caring · Care ethics · Patient involvement · Patient perspective · Epistemic injustice · Inclusion

T. Teunissen (✉)
Leyden Academy and the University of Humanistic Studies, Leiden, The Netherlands

T. Abma
Leiden University Medical Centre, Leiden, The Netherlands

1   Introduction

This chapter is about my journey from getting a chronic illness and with the accompanying stamp "patient" slowly move toward "researcher with lived experience." For a number of years, I have been involved on a voluntary basis as a researcher at the university and at a knowledge institute where I do research on the inclusive and just society. Over the years, despite as well as thanks to my health problems, I have miraculously ended up there. This story tells about that and about my quest: how can I contribute to the realization of meaningful, just and structural patient participation and the introduction of the patient's perspective?

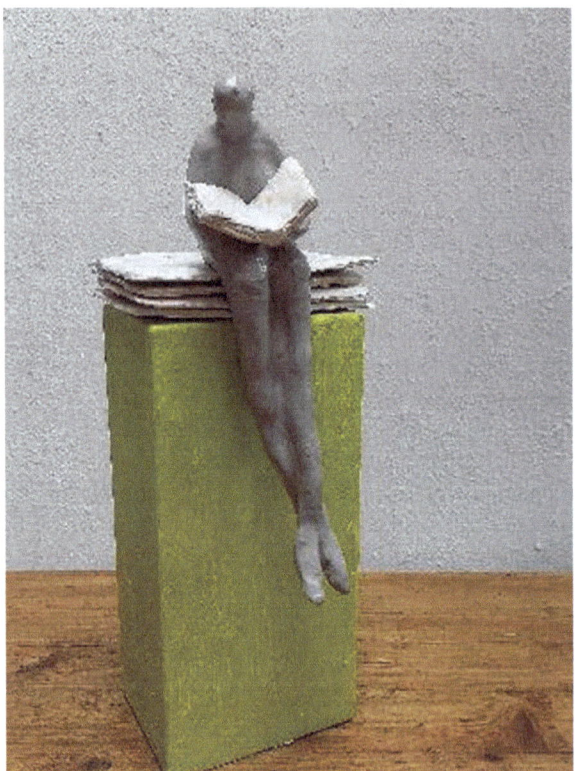

Reading, reading, reading (Teunissen, 2022)

Reading, reading, reading (Teunissen et al. 2019)

The story is constructed according to Denzin (2014) autoethnographic method and divided into episodes (Heisel et al. 2016). The draft text was drawn up in Dutch and then translated into English.

I use two story lines in the chapter; my journey from patient to researcher with lived experience and the story of my 3-weekly infusion, a treatment I need for my primary immuno deficiency (PID). Both stories are about obstacles and dilemmas in my life. The two stories run parallel along the themes: illness experience and moti-vation, key moments (McAdams 2001), motivation to become a researcher with lived experience, meaningful experience, support and lessons learned. Finally, in a short reflection I look at the meaning of living with chronic conditions and becom-ing a patient researcher for my life. The texts in blue italics are about an infu-sion day.

> 07:30 a.m.: This morning upon getting up I knew immediately, another infusion today. Even though this has been the situation every three weeks for over a year now, I still feel a slight tension rising, a somewhat restless feeling… Would it go well this time… do I inject right the first time or do I have to do it again? Those kinds of things. Hopefully the infusion pump alarm won't go off again like last time because then I'll immediately be shocked and I have to call the online nurses with trembling fingers about what to do. I feel very unsafe at such a moment with the needle in my body connected to an IV and an alarm bell that keeps going off… it is difficult for me not to panic completely. Well, the district nurses assured me the previous times on the phone that I was really not in any danger… Still, I would rather have the infusions take place in the hospital, like the first three times. From the 4th time, the district nurse did it at home to teach me. After 10 infusions they wanted to stop this home support, apparently because it is too expensive, as it turned out when asked, and I had to do it myself. Except in special cases, they said… If people are alone, we will keep coming, the nurse told us or if people are chaotic or very emotional during the IV insertion. Then they—always very emphatically—said to me "You are doing well, and you can do it very well yourself!" That normally sounds like a compliment. It didn't feel like that now.

2 Core of the Illness Experience and Motivation

2.1 From One-Time to Chronic

I think back to how it all started. In 1984 we moved our family with two small chil-dren to another part of the country where we had bought an old house that needed to be renovated. After half a year of renovation, the problems started. I got pneumo-nia for the first time in my life and thought: "after a good summer with a lot of being outside and resting, then it will be over." The hopes and expectations that this was an incident, a one-off, turned out to be wrong. The pneumonias recurred and after several lung examinations I was diagnosed with asthma, a chronic lung disease. I was very shocked by that because it meant that it would not end with 1 bad year with chronic lung problems. The word "lifelong" flashed through my mind briefly. But—who knows—things will turn out differently for me. The periods of being sick, recovering and being healthy again alternated. The healthy periods became shorter and shorter. When two rare chronic diseases were added over the years (eye cancer and a primary immune disorder), I lost my courage. I only felt like a patient, I had become the disease. I realized and experienced with my head, heart, and body that chronic diseases had become a permanent thing that I had to continue to take into account, privately but also in my work, in my social life, with my hobbies; in short, literally everything I did.

2.2 From Me to We

When it dawned on me that this situation remained, I tried to fit this into my life as best I could. But I also started to wonder how the other 1.6 million Dutch people with one or more chronic illnesses deal with the problems in their work and social lives that result from this. I wonder how they keep their spirits up as they keep falling over and over and then working hard to get back up, knowing they will fall again soon. The pattern repeats itself. What did these people like me find meaningful in their life (giving meaning)? Then I saw a vacancy for someone on a patient advisory board. I applied and became a board member. I decided to commit myself not only for myself but for the group of people with chronic illnesses. Over the following years I became involved in patient councils of health funds, patient associations, advisory committees, became a patient expert in research projects, became co-researcher and board member of a national umbrella organization that represents the interests of people with a chronic illness or disability

> 08:00 a.m.: Well, let's not get ahead of things and start to get the infusion fluid out of the fridge so it's up to temperature when I start the infusion tonight. Making my breakfast, that's the first thing I'm going to do now.

3 Justice and Inclusion, Pseudo Participation, and Meaningful Participation

Often, when I was asked again to introduce the patient perspective into a plan, project or research, together with other people with a chronic illness, we got stuck in the process. We asked ourselves: Patient perspective, how, then where, what then? What exactly is the patient perspective? What is important here? What are the ethical dilemmas of/for patients with this proposal? Do we actually know what people in our patient group consider urgent or important? And the patients you don't hear or who don't make themselves heard—the "silent" patients—then, we don't just want to look after the interests of the empowered patients, do we? I was committed to not excluding people and I wanted to try to do justice to the voices of people with illness whether they speak loudly and loudly or whisper or even remain silent. It shouldn't be who is silent consents and slogans like that. The opinion of people with a disease counts, they are carriers of knowledge about living with the disease and the problems that arise from it. I have often experienced that I or fellow sufferers were not taken seriously or that the reliability of our story was doubted. Prejudices about patients—they are emotional, they have not learned for this profession—play a role in this. Fricker (2007), an English philosopher, used the term "epistemic injustice" for this. People who don't raise their voices loudly are often not believed. If they express themselves differently than the "norm," their message will not be recognized or acknowledged. In the eyes of researchers, politicians or people with power in important positions in society, they are "just" patients, so what could they know about the subject?

In the meantime, I noticed that the perspective of patients was hardly introduced, let alone that anything was done with it in practice, in healthcare projects, in health research, and in policy. I thought this had to be done differently, better, but above all fairer. It turned out to be difficult and frustrating for any of us patients to bring in the patient perspective. And when we put in our points, they listened politely but didn't do much with it in the end. The terms "pseudo participation" and "tokenism" became more and more a reality. But giving up was not an option, I thought, because the perspective of patients had to be brought in, that was a matter of justice. After all, patients were the target group for which the services or products such as medicines were developed. The bottlenecks and needs of patients should be the starting point and the focal point of a care inquiry and not as a side issue or irrelevant. They are the relevant stakeholders in research that is about patients, in my opinion. The book "Nothing About Us Without Us" by Charlton (2000) was an indictment of the oppression of disabilities, which he says are rooted in degradation, dependence, and powerlessness. This is experienced in one form or another by 500 million people across the world with physical, sensory, cognitive or developmental disabilities. I embrace the slogan "nothing about us without us" and this became my motto.

4   My Quest

Gradually, I not only tried to get us to sit down and take part as patients in committees or in projects, but I went one step further. I tried to develop the preconditions for structural meaningful patient participation in which patients are equal discussion partners in all phases of a research or project. My main goal became to develop scientifically substantiated preconditions and tools together with and for patients. It was important that these would be recognized and accepted by the patient world and seen by the scientific world as reliable and solidly substantiated. I decided to take it as my personal "quest," a quest for how the patient perspective could be better introduced, and how it could be more meaningful, more structural, more inclusive and fairer. To realize this, I started a PhD trajectory, and these became the questions to be investigated in my PhD research (Teunissen 2014).

08:45 a.m.: I check my cell phone and see my girlfriend is asking if I'm coming for coffee tonight. Just answer that tonight it won't work because it's my infusion day. Tomorrow is a visit to my in-laws. They are already very old and live in Brabant. I hope the side effects of the infusion, which sometimes last up to 24 h, are not too bad this time. Then I feel like I have the flu, my body aches and I'm feverish. Hoping it goes well this time. My in-laws clearly have a need for contact, but they also want to "make a difference" by already bringing cake with the coffee in the house for when we come and want to pamper us and take care of us. Sometimes they don't see or speak to anyone for days. Loneliness is lurking… we have to pay close attention to that as family, in-laws and children. It remains a bottleneck: how do I take care of others when my health is an obstacle and is so erratic?

5   Key Concepts of My Patient Experience Are: Meaningful Experience

One of the key concepts of my patient experience is the more erratic aspect of having a chronic illness. The capriciousness of the disease remains difficult to deal with for myself but also for those around me. If I have to cancel another birthday and get questions like: "or do you not feel like it or something?" In good periods I do everything, and I also plan everything for work, hobby, sports, birthday parties, outings. I don't want to just sit around and wait until I get ill, but to start living and the moment I get ill again I step on the brake. No fun and always a bit sad, those cancel phone calls "oh yeah dude? Ill again? … Get well soon." Wishing you to get well soon is nice—empathizing with the other is very important—but the feeling also creeps up on me. I'll be better soon, but for how long? I wonder what my mindset or attitude toward myself and others should be; always sick and patient or am I healthy, a whole person and sometimes ill? Annoying.

Incomprehension is another key concept and a recurring thing. My social environment is sometimes full of incomprehension: "I saw you cycling yesterday and now you feel ill…," "I don't see anything about you, are you really ill?" The fact that you have a disease but are not always ill remains difficult to understand for those around me, but sometimes also for myself. What also plays into this is that you usually cannot see a chronic illness—in contrast to a disability that can often be seen from the outside. You don't miss an arm or sit in a wheelchair. Trust and credibility are important components that play a role in the interaction between patients and their environment. If at times my illness does not bother me much, I make appointments (too) enthusiastically, plan activities or take on obligations. But then reality kicks in after days or weeks and I have to unsubscribe again. Finding a balance in this for myself and toward others is a recurring struggle.

Finally, another important key concept from my decades of patient experience, and even to this day I must confess, is the dilemma of having a disease or being a disease. I have a chronic illness but am not always feeling ill. One day I can't do something, the next I can. I don't want to narrow down my identity, the person that I am, to my illness. I am more than my illness, I am a human being, a versatile person with certain character traits, convictions, norms, and values—with which I want to engage the world and my environment. For example, in my life I often experience a struggle between wanting and having to take care of myself, but also want to take care of others at the same time. I want to belong as a person in society, in my work, in my family and circle of friends, in my reading club. I don't want to be solely defined or reduced to a disease. I want to participate in society, but above all I want to matter and be of significance to others.

6   The Motivation to Become a Researcher as a Patient

As a PhD student and later as a scientific researcher, I developed a list of criteria and values together with other patients. This tool is used in realizing the patient perspective in committees and platforms and in assessments and evaluations of project proposals in health research and healthcare from the patient perspective by patients and their representatives. After 12 years, this criteria list is still in use in many places in the Netherlands.

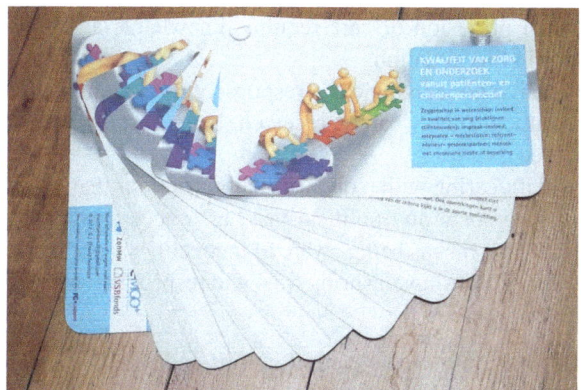

2013 The first criteria fan

2013 The first criteria fan

I do not only want to reduce or solve the bottlenecks and dilemmas that arise due to the disease(s) and living with the disease(s) for myself, but I want to work on reducing this for the entire patient group. My motivation is to also take care of the others with a disease through action research. I want to help make the voice of the group of people with a disease heard loud and clear. I also want to do justice to the "silent patients," the people who for whatever reason can't make their voice heard or whisper. Acknowledging and recognizing what their experiences are (Fricker 2007). I want to collect their bottlenecks, concerns, and values from them and make them count in policy, research, and care practice. These ideas are in line with the ideas of a caring society in which trust and solidarity are the pillars.

I agree with the ideas and theories about care and care ethics of Tronto (1993, 2013) where she sees care as a cyclical process in which five phases of care are discussed, for which you need different core values or ethically good manners. In addition to caring about, caring that, providing care, receiving care—this also includes worrying. Seeing care as both a personal and political task, as a necessary practice to promote social equality, based on justice, equality, and freedom for all. Tronto (1993, 2013) explains five core values of concern in her books: attention, responsibility, competence, responsiveness, and solidarity. Care is also a universal human need that is necessary in order to function and it is, therefore, not only vulnerable people in our society who need care and also people who need care want to be able to care/look after the other; this is important for every person.

1. Phase caring about/caring about (attention): Moral actions that go with it: Becoming aware of the care demand, having an eye for recognizing what the care need is.
2. Phase taking care/ensuring that (responsibility): Moral actions that go with it You feel responsible, and someone has to take responsibility (apply for it) for the identified care demand. Can it be allowed in the given context.
3. Phase care giving/providing care (competence): moral actions that are part of this: The actual provision of care requires knowledge and competence. What care is needed in this situation.
4. Phase care receiving/receiving care (responsiveness) moral actions that go with it. Paying attention to how care is received, being responsive and being able to adapt where necessary.
5. Phase caring with/caring with (solidarity) moral actions that go with it are seeing care as both a personal and political task, as a necessary practice to promote social equality. This means being aware of inequalities, conflicts and vulnerabilities in the care relationship, ensuring trust and respect between the care provider and the care recipient.

By doing research I try to take care of myself and to look after others in accordance with these five care phases and to ensure a more just and inclusive society together with others. I try to work inspired by the ideas from the ethics of care and of a caring society that deal with the basic questions such as "What should I do?" and "What is the good life?". I am guided by values such as involvement, dependence, responsibility, vulnerability, respect, inclusion, and openness (Visse and Abma 2018; Heijst 2008; Leget 2013).

10.00 a.m.: Oh just remembered: I always have to check whether the infusion liquid is not cloudy but clear … otherwise it cannot be used and I have to order new liquid at the pharmacy … but that will take at least two days before I have that in the house … Fortunately the liquid is clear and I also see that I have one more in stock in the fridge. I feel lucky. I'm fine today.

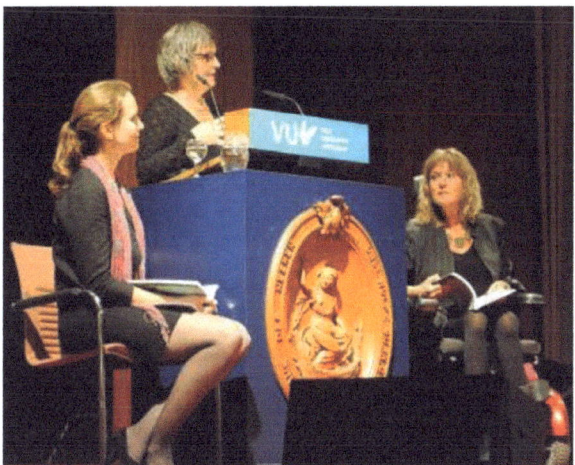

2014 Defending my thesis at the VU-University in Amsterdam

2014 Defending my thesis at the VU-University in Amsterdam

From the period before my research as a PhD, and until today, I have been involved as a member of various program committees of the Dutch organization for health research and development ZonMW. My areas of focus are meaningful patient or citizen participation (PPi), inclusion, e-justice, and care ethics. After a period as a policy officer at a large national patient organization, I was then given the opportunity, to my great surprise, but with even more joy, to do scientific research in this area as a PhD. This allowed me to do research based on the ideas of care, care ethics with special attention to justice and inclusion. I focused, in close collaboration with the patient field, on developing practical patient criteria and values as a tool for patient participation (the "criteria range"). This made bringing in the perspective of patients more doable for patients and their representatives. It gave them support and structure. Also, working with six patient criteria and values over and over again gave the perspective of patients a more serious place in research, policy agendas, and in decision-making in health research, healthcare or in committees. After my PhD on these topics, I became a social science researcher.

Nowadays, participation, social justice, and inclusion are the core themes in my work as a researcher. Unfortunately, I will always remain a person with chronic illnesses, often referred to as a patient, often dependent on relatives, care providers, treatments, and medication. But also, an additional dimension has been added by targeting and developing myself as a researcher with lived experience. I explicitly use my patient experience in my research work. I even choose topics for research and write about them that have common ground with chronic illness, including my own illness experience, such as: illness and meaning; meaning full of life with illness; art and care; meaningful patient participation.

10:20 a.m.: I drink a cup of coffee and decide to prepare dinner on time. We will eat early, my husband Paul already knows that. Then I can start with the infusion afterwards and watch a movie sitting on the couch when the IV is connected and running. After two hours

I can disconnect everything and collapse relieved on the couch for another hour of being free ... with nothing I must do ... being loose and able to move. This is an important moment because I have fought back to keep the disease small again for the next three weeks. I still have an influence on what happens to me.

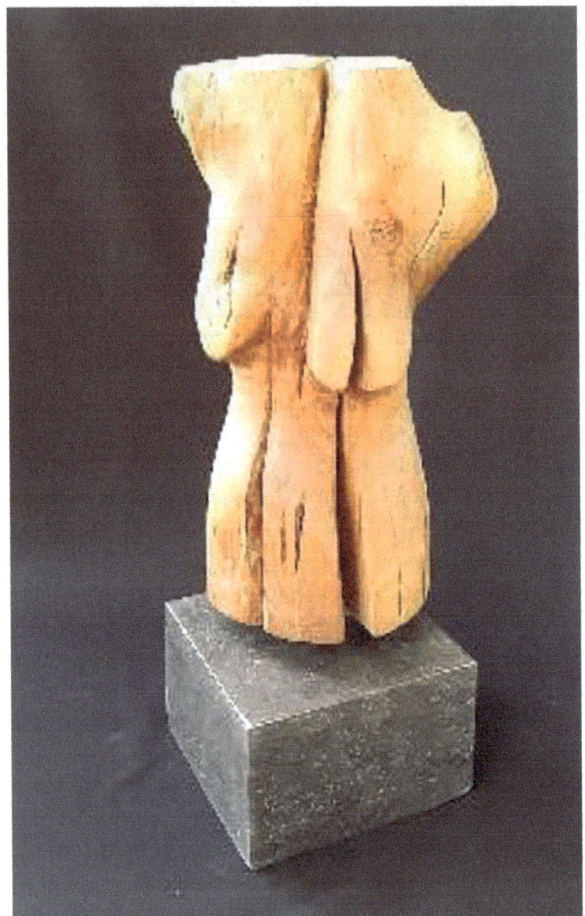

Lived through (Teunissen, 2003)

Lived through (Teunissen 2014)

But the dark side of my work as a researcher is that due to my illnesses, the research work regularly stagnates, or I must reschedule appointments, or I can't attend meetings. It also remains difficult after a period of illness to re-join the ongoing process. You actually have to sprint to make up for the overdue time and work, but of course that only partially succeeds because the energy is limited after a period of illness. That remains difficult and I regularly doubt whether it is not better for my environment if I no longer take on any tasks and obligations at all to prevent this period of being ill and not being able to join in again soon. But I like it too much and still have the idea that I can mean something to others in this way. I'll just take the hiccups for now. Because doing research and writing about it is meaningful to me; it gives voice to my experiences, I am being heard and read. I am giving insight into the lived experience, testifying about living with illnesses. Yet I no longer experience my illness experience as just a burden but can now also use it constructively by drawing attention to the issues and needs of other patients and where possible improving the situation for them through research and writing. As a result, to my own surprise, I have become an expert with both professional and experiential knowledge. And that greatly softens the often-daily struggle and toil that the illnesses entail for me.

6.1   The Most Meaningful Experience as a Patient Researcher

One of my most meaningful experiences as a researcher with lived experience is that together with people with illness or disability I have developed a set of criteria and values that makes it easier for people who participate in a committee or in a research team to introduce the patient perspective. In practice, this set functions as a tool for people that bring the patient's perspective to the table in committees, platforms or consultative councils. I find it particularly valuable to experience that this tool—which now has all kinds of versions, various designs and contents for various target groups—is still used in practice after 12 years and that there is still a demand for it to this day. Apparently, this tool works in practice. I also experience it as particularly meaningful to write and publish scientific articles about dilemmas and bottlenecks in my life with diseases, using the autoethnographic method. In the articles I place my own dilemmas and bottlenecks during living with multiple diseases, next to theories and the current social discourse and reflect on them. These articles are about the struggle and strength for living with illness, about living a meaningful life by also being able to care for others and about continuing to love in addition to receiving care. They are still regularly quoted, and I still get questions to come and talk about this (Teunissen 2014; Teunissen et al. 2015, 2018, 2019).

> 11.15 p.m.: I am walking in town and suddenly I get an alarming feeling: did I charge the battery of the infusion pump last time? Oops not checked…. When I get home, must do it immediately so that I can still charge the battery in time, because that takes a few hours. My strolling around in shops immediately seems time-wasting and pointless. I hurry to find my bike and go home. I don't want to think about the battery being empty in the middle of the infusion and the hassle with needles and tubing if that were suddenly happening … the whole thing would take even more time…. Have to pay more attention next time.

I am providing insight into the lived experience, testifying about living with illnesses, stories countering the policies and projections of others. The personal has become political and also stands for Tronto's 5th stage of care: caring with. Little is written about being ill, both in the literature and in scientific literature. Woolf (1930) already made this observation when she wrote the essay "On being ill." Anyone who is ill, she writes, is cut off from the world. The patient lies in bed while the "army of the standing" marches on. He who is healthy "gets ready for battle," the ill one is the "deserter." So why, Woolf wonders, isn't being ill in literature on a par with "love, fight, and jealousy" and all those other things that shrug off the familiar perspective. Why are there no "novels written about the flu, epic poems about typhoid, lyrics about toothache?" And that observation seems to be still valid in 2022. In literature, increasingly more stories about illness experiences appear, such as those published by Marsman (2018) and Zonneveld (2020). Currently, there are only sporadic stories about illness experiences in scientific literature. There are many patient experience stories, but these do not have the characteristics of literature or scientific literature. Usually, they are a piece of narrative text to illustrate a story about the medical treatment or the cause of the disease. In the Netherlands, for example, there is a still growing collection of more than 6000 experience stories from patients and their relatives, which is managed by Erasmus Universiteit (2022). Patients, relatives, citizens, researchers, policy makers, and other professionals can make use of this.

6.2 Experienced Support

During my journey I have experienced a lot of support from other people with a chronic illness or disability who are committed to introducing the patient or client perspective in care and welfare practice, in research and in policy, the so-called experience experts or patient experts. Partners in crime that's how it felt. We stand up and draw attention to not being heard as a group and want to have a say and influence and be recognized as a relevant equal partner in discussions. But of course, I experienced a lot of support from my family when I was ill on the couch again, but I gave my scarce energy that day to want to introduce patients' perspective in a committee or a research project.

Living with chronic diseases often means living with limited energy, with energy depleted in the middle of the day and exhaustion ensuing. Going to bed an hour earlier, something healthy people do when tired, will not work. This limited energy means always having to compromise and weigh things up, not to a birthday, not out shopping in the city with my daughter for a new coat or not to a reception or to a meeting. Support and understanding from my family and loved ones are extremely important and even indispensable.

> 17:30 p.m.: Dinner is ready. After dinner I'm about to start. First, I have to put on other loose-fitting clothes because a pair of jeans with a belt does not work with the needle and tube of the IV in my abdomen. Then I get the IV stuff together and also the note with the 14 consecutive steps that I have to go through. A few moments later it is ready, there are two glasses of water, hot tea and there are some cookies on the table next to the TV remote and the telephone. The movie is ready to play. All I have to do is press the IV pump start button. During my journey, both as a patient with lived experience, and now on the couch with the infusion, I often had to bite the bullet to eventually achieve an improvement.

6.3   Learned Lessons

Being a researcher with lived experience has taught me a number of lessons about motivation, serious participation, preconditions, being taken seriously, and about ethical work.

My motivation in doing research has to do with "taking care of others" in which topics such as epistemic injustice, exclusion, and working on meaningful patient participation are the core values. Questions about what a good life is for people with disabilities and how to live a meaningful life despite health problems are also worth attention and research. Focusing by staying close to these causes and values is important to me especially in the context of illness and associated limited energy. In my view, the following three arguments apply to the subject of patient participation to justify the participation of patients in decision-making regarding scientific research (Abma and Broerse 2007):

Normative argument: As end users of the results of the research, patients have the right to knowledge exchange, having a say and taking part in decision-making.

Substantive argument: Patients are the "experts by experience" in dealing with the disease in all domains of life; this is relevant for the purpose, design, and implementation of the research.

Political argument: patient participation leads to more support for research because it is more in line with the wishes and needs of patients. It also stimulates the implementation and early availability of new treatment methods.

Control: The organization of people with a chronic illness or disability is the principal and has full control of content

Partnership: People with a chronic illness or disability cooperate as equal partners with other parties and take decisions jointly

Advice: People with a chronic illness or disability offer advice when asked but take no group decisions

Consultation: People with a chronic illness or disability are asked for their opinion

No participation: People with a chronic illness or disability do not ask and are not asked

Another important precondition for me to work or talk about patient participation in research, for example, is that the researcher gives the patient a clear and serious role with tasks and authorities in advance. A patient or an experience expert can be involved in various ways with various roles and tasks in research or policy or in projects (see Fig. 1). But there are also preconditions that are of crucial importance to patient participation. Together with Wit et al. (2016) I have made an inventory of these preconditions.

These concern, respectively:

Phase patients should participate in multiple phases of research;
Role of the patient—Integration of the patient perspective in scientific research requires a combination of different forms of participation, on several steps of the participation ladder;

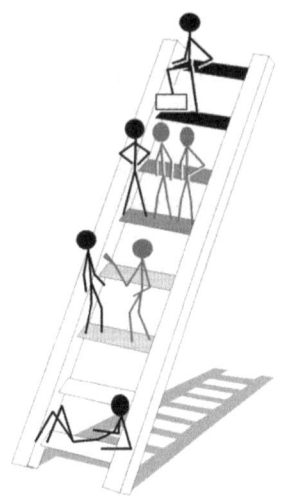

Control The organization of people with a chronic illness or disability is the principal and has full control of content

Partnership People with a chronic illness or disability cooperate as equal partners with other parties and take decisions jointly

Advice People with a chronic illness or disability offer advice when asked but take no group decisions

Consultation People with a chronic illness or disability are asked for their opinion

No participation People with a chronic illness or disability do not ask and are not asked

© G.J.Teunissen

Fig. 1 Patient participation ladder (Teunissen 2014)

Recruitment and selection—The recruitment of patient representatives should be supported by a clear job description (profile) and a recruitment strategy with attention to diversity and representativeness;

Support—Patient representatives should receive tailor-made information and coaching, both through a good introduction at the start and during the study;

Financing—Patient participation costs money and should be budgeted realistically. Expenses of patient representatives must be reimbursed:

Training—Training for both patient representatives and researchers benefits scientific research. Prior to any research in which patients participate, the need for training should be discussed with those involved;

Evaluation—The contributions of patient representatives to the research and the collaboration with the researchers should be regularly evaluated;

Making visible—The form of participation and the contributions of patient representatives should be carefully described. The method of publication is the subject of discussion between researchers and patient representatives;

Recognition—The contribution of patient representatives should be appropriately acknowledged both during and after a trial.

6.4   Ethics, Inclusion, and Fairness

But it is also important to me with patient participation that during the research the (raw, pure) experience is collected of the large group of patients who do not participate in the research. This has to do with ethics, inclusion and justice, including epistemic justice. This can often be done in collaboration with the patient association. Therefore, experience should not come only from the assertive patient who gives his opinion. Rather researchers should be—actively—looking for (a sample) of patients in the country who might not complete an online survey and not participate in platforms or councils. Collecting the experience with the disease of these people too, allows taking it into account in the research. A researcher should always think about patient participation: e.g., who am I not hearing, which parts of the patient group are not participating in these interviews or in this focus group. That too is ethical work in research: who do I exclude and who am I not reaching?

> 18.00 p.m.: Every time I have to overcome something to stick the IV needle in my abdomen. Fumbling with small stickers, caps, closing clips. Dose the first "place making" liquid with a separate syringe in small bits through the tube and the needle in my abdomen using a stopwatch. Then wait exactly eight minutes before another tube can be connected to the needle. Then the infusion pump can be switched on to infuse the second liquid with the immunoglobulins. These compensate for the missing part of my immune system and last some three weeks. I have to stay calm when the pump gives an alarm when there is an air bubble. I practice patience, hear sounds, see hoses, am sitting still, keep watching if there is no bleeding. I am focusing on what I am doing and always keep an eye on my goal. This remains important, whether it's carefully running my IV or working on a social problem.

6.5   Be Alert to not Being Taken Seriously

People with experiential knowledge can contribute their experience and knowledge about what it means to live with the disease every day and what consequences this has in all areas of life such as health education, work, leisure, mobility, education, social contacts. Which dilemmas arise and which obstacles. Professionals have acquired professional knowledge during their training and during their work on a specific subject or field and they know, for example, the guidelines and the protocols.

Together, experiential knowledge and professional knowledge complement each other very nicely. By entering into such a partnership, a solid foundation is created, so that a study or a project or guideline becomes diverse, richer, and more reliable and that it has a greater chance of a better result and a better connection with the practical situation. It should be or become an intrinsic need and motivation of a researcher to also conduct research about people with people themselves. But professional knowledge and experiential knowledge can also clash and lead to conflict. This clash is already caused by the fact that you as patient(s) are not always taken seriously. In short, your experience as a patient is either recognized as meaningful and relevant input or not. The words you might choose to say something can deviate from the professional jargon and are, therefore, not given a proper place in the minutes of meeting, reports or documents. This is what Fricker (2007) calls such not recognizing and acknowledging the patients' knowledge "epistemic injustice."

"Nothing about us without us" should become the norm and realizing a patient's perspective in all phases of research or project should become part of the researcher's moral toolbox. This is of vital importance to me and it is the core of patient participation. Doing research with the people themselves is not something you add at the end. It requires "ethical work" (Groot-Sluijsmans 2021) in which co-ownership, collaboration, and shared decision-making are at the core. Banks and Nøhr (2013) coined the term "ethics work" from social work. Groot and Abma (2022) translated this to the field of research with patients. They refer to the invisible work you do as a researcher to care for and build relationships with people when you do research with them. A part of ethical work is "relation work," connecting people, aligning people. Doing good research is not only according to existing scientific research methods, but also ethically good participatory research. When conducting research with people and for people, the perspectives of the people themselves—in this case people with a chronic illness—should be the basis and starting point in the research, as well as the participation of a group of patients during the research in a role as an equal partner.

Finally, I still work as a scientific guest researcher on a voluntary basis - because a regular paid permanent job is not possible due to the capriciousness of the diseases. I combine scientific knowledge and experiential knowledge, as researching and understanding these issues is of the utmost importance to make progress. Writing remains meaningful to me; give voice to my experiences, be heard and my writing being read. It allows me to provide insight into the lived experience, to testify about living with illnesses, and to counter the policies and projections of others. My journey of becoming a researcher after many years with lived experience as well as my three-weekly infusion day trip are far from over but will continue unabated: there is still a lot of work to be done.

> 18:45 p.m.: I am finally sitting on the couch with lots of pillows around me, the IV is plugged in and the IV pump is making a familiar humming noise. Water and a second cup of tea are within reach. I'm watching the movie. The pump stays quiet this time, no alarm bells or anything. After an hour or two the IV fluid has run into my body, I can start disconnecting everything. Removing the stuck-on needle in particular remains painful. Then safely store the needle in the needle container. Make sure I don't prick myself at the last minute, it hurts viciously. And then back on the couch, free of the hose, pump and needle. Hope I get three quiet boring weeks as far as the illnesses are concerned….

6.6   Reflection (by Prof. Dr. Tineke Abma)

Truus has asked me to write a short reflection, and I really like to do that. For readers it is good to know that Truus and I have known each other since 2010. She obtained her PhD with me and was associated with the university where I was a professor for many years. She is currently affiliated with the Leyden Academy on Vitality and Aging, of which I am an Executive-Director, besides my professorship at Leiden University Medical Centre.

In this chapter Truus combines two storylines: the story of the daily struggle with the chronic disease and the story of the patient who transforms into a researcher. It provides a phenomenological insight into the illness experience from a first-person perspective, demonstrating that the illness experience is a rich source of knowledge for the patient researcher. That is also what Truus advocates: use the "raw" experiences of illness, as expressed in the story about the infusion pump, with the feelings of fear and panic that the alarm will go off, the idea that you have to be self-sufficient and the concern that if that doesn't work, you may not be a good patient in the eyes of policy makers, and all the illness work you have to do, let those experiences resonate in your role as a researcher. I think that is an important message, because patient researchers can also become alienated from their own personal experiences, and—unconsciously—censor them, because they do not fit in with the expert role of researcher and the academic context where distance and objectivity are the norm.

We can link this phenomenon of alienation and proto-professionalization to the power dynamics and hierarchy of knowledge. Personal experiences are suspect in a scientific context because they are considered subjective. However, it is precisely this subjectivity, the personal experience, and the insider perspective that is of added value for scientific researchers. A professional will first and foremost approach a sick patient by looking at the disease, viewing that disease from the outside as a matter of establishing a diagnosis and treatment. However, the patient approaches the illness as a disruption in the biography and focuses on the meaning and experience of the illness. These are two completely different and therefore complementary, and sometimes conflicting, perspectives.

Conflicting, because a patient demands attention for the personal life situation as a person and the meaning of the illness, while the professional mainly searches for a solution for the disease. It is therefore crucial that a patient researcher is constantly encouraged to share these subjective experiences, to witness and relate about the illness experiences, and that a context is created in which that experience can be there, even if they are raw, chaotic, emotional, and subjective. The witnessing and sense making contribute to epistemic justice in the field of healthcare (Carel and Kidd 2014), and in healthcare research (Groot et al. 2022).

Witnessing and being heard is meaningful for the patient researcher. Likewise, for me as a professor it is always good and enriching to hear Truus' story. Her first-person account forms a reality check and helps me to see what patients encounter and what research should focus on. Moreover, these experiences correct my tendency as a professional to think in simple solutions and quick fixes.

References

Abma TA, Broerse J. Zeggenschap in wetenschap. Patiëntenparticipatie in theorie en praktijk. [Having a say in science. Patient involvement in theory and practice]. Den Haag: LEMMA; 2007.

Banks S, Nøhr K, editors. Practicing social work ethics around the world: cases and commentaries. London: Routledge; 2013.

Carel H, Kidd IJ. Epistemic injustice in healthcare: a philosophical analysis. Med Health Care Philos. 2014;17:529–40.

Charlton JI. Nothing about us without us: disability, empowerment and oppression. Univ Calif Press. 2000;19:1075–80.

Denzin NK. Interpretive autoethnography. Los Angeles: Sage; 2014.

Erasmus Universiteit. Patient ervaringsverhalen. [Patient experience stories]. 2022. https://www.patientervaringsverhalen.nl/. Accessed 30 August 2022.

Fricker M. Epistemic injustice: power and the ethics of knowing. Oxford: University Press; 2007.

Groot B, Abma T. Ethics framework for citizen science and public and patient participation in research. BMC Med Ethics. 2022;23:1–9.

Groot B, Haveman A, Abma T. Relational, ethically sound co-production in mental health care research: epistemic injustice and the need for an ethics of care. Crit Public Health. 2022;32:230–40.

Groot-Sluijsmans BC. Ethics of participatory health research: insights from a reflective journey. Doctoral dissertation, VU Amsterdam. Alblasserdam, Ridderprint. 2021.

Heijst A. Iemand zien staan; Zorgethiek over erkenning. [To see somebody. Care ethics about acknowledging]. Kampen: Uitgeverij Klement; 2008.

Heisel MJ, Neufeld E, Flett GL. Reasons for living, meaning in life, and suicide ideation: investigating the roles of key positive psychological factors in reducing suicide risk in community-residing older adults. Aging Ment Health. 2016;20(2):195–207. https://doi.org/10.1080/13607863.2015.1078279.

Leget C. Analyzing dignity: a perspective from the ethics of care. Med Health Care Philos. 2013;16:945–52.

Marsman L. Hoe gaat het met je? De scan duurt vijf minuten. [How are you? The scan takes five minutes]. Amsterdam: Uitgeverij Pluim; 2018.

McAdams DP. The psychology of life stories. Rev Gen Psychol. 2001;5:100–22.

Teunissen GJ. Values and criteria of people with chronic illness or disability. Doctoral dissertation, VU Amsterdam. 2014.

Teunissen GJ, Visse MA, Abma TA. Struggling between strength and vulnerability, a patients' counter story. Health Care Anal. 2015;23:288–305.

Teunissen GJ, Lindhout P, Abma TA. Balancing loving and caring in times of chronic illness. Qual Res J. 2018;18:210–22.

Teunissen T, Lindhout P, Schipper K, Abma T. Living a meaningful life and taking good care of oneself in times of illness: highlighting a dilemma. IJFAB. 2019;12:44–60.

Tronto JC. Moral boundaries: a political argument for an ethic of care. New York: Psychology Press; 1993.

Tronto JC. Caring democracy markets, equality and justice. New York: University Press; 2013.

Visse MA, Abma TA. Evaluation for a caring society. San Bernardino: IAP Publishers; 2018.

Wit M, Bloemkolk D, Teunissen T, van Rensen A. Voorwaarden voor succesvolle patiënten / cliënten betrokkenheid bij medisch biomedisch onderzoek. [Conditions for successful patient/client involvement in medical biomedical research]. TSG. 2016;94:91–100.

Woolf V. On being ill. Richmond: Hogarth Press; 1930.

Zonneveld M. Gods ruïne. [God's ruin]. Amsterdam: Uitgeverij Het Moet; 2020.

Is Doctor Google our Best Choice for Healthcare Information Recommendations? A Duty of Care to Improve Processes

Frada Burstein and Grant Meredith

Abstract Living with a life-long medical condition or a serious disease requires a lot of research skills on how to access the best quality information to inform better decision-making of healthcare consumers. Relatives, friends, and carers are often sharing the stress and responsibility of looking after the healthcare of consumers. They feel personally responsible for meeting not only physical, but also information needs of people they care for. With the internet being almost a default source of a wide variety of information, and health information in particular, this interview-based chapter reflects on what are the opportunities and challenges for information and communication technology (ICT) researchers who aim to address the personalized needs for quality healthcare information provision.

Professor Frada Burstein is a leading information technology researcher specializing in smart information portals in health care. Her research has contributed to the transformations in web-based information systems architecture to empower patients. She was named the ICT Educator of the Year for her pioneering work in knowledge management and ICT education. In this interview with Grant Meredith, she reveals how her intense experiences caring for her father led her to focus her intelligent systems research toward health care.

Keywords Personalized healthcare · Digital repositories · Information needs

F. Burstein (✉)
Department of Human Centred Computing, Faculty of Information Technology, Monash University, Melbourne, VIC, Australia
e-mail: frada.burstein@monash.edu

G. Meredith
Global Professional School, Federation University, Ballarat, VIC, Australia

A. Stranieri et al. (eds.), *Research Partners with Lived Experience*,
https://doi.org/10.1007/978-981-97-0033-2_7

1   Researcher and Carer

Grant: Can you tell me a little bit about yourself, maybe like your education, where did you grow up? What is your profession or your past professions, etc., please.

Frada: I grew up in Georgia in the former Soviet Union. We moved to Australia just before the Soviet Union collapsed and we came as a family with my husband and two children as skilled migrants in the early 90s. I had done my PhD in computer science effectively in decision support systems at the Institute of Cybernetics in Tbilisi which was at the Georgian Academy of Sciences, a part of the USSR Academy of Sciences. I've been working in research ever since then.

When I finished my PhD. I started working in that same institute in the laboratory that was researching decision support systems of all sorts. I was doing decision support systems research with various organisations, including Georgian archeologists which was part of my PhD as well.

So, I was very interested in the "human side" of computer systems and computer programs. That's what brought me to information systems research effectively because we did not quite have that recognised as a specific discipline at the time, My PhD was actually in Technical Cybernetics and Information Theory. So, it had a lot of maths in it. But as I mentioned already, in my doctoral research I proposed new algorithms, but I was more interested in how they could be implemented to help people make better decisions.

After a couple of years, we were settled in Australia, and my parents arrived. They didn't intend to stay, but my father was involved in a very bad car accident just a couple of weeks before they had to leave. He was struck by a car and became a quadriplegic. From that point onward my "carer" journey began. I was in and out of hospitals with him for 14 years, and I observed first-hand how doctors had been dealing with information systems. As a result, over time, I began to truly appreciate how badly they were being supported by technology. I remember hearing a senior surgeon saying that when he is in the operating theater, he feels like he's in the twenty-first century, but when he's back at his office computer, it's the nineteenth century.

These interactions with medical professionals really opened my eyes. I was interested in learning yet another side of technology. I was still interested in, what the problems were that people have with using technology effectively to seek information for effective decision-making. As a result of caring for my father, I noted that medicine and clinical practice is where you can see those deficiencies at a very high, but also practical level. So that's how the notion of being a "reflective researcher" became and still is, really close to my heart. As decision support systems researchers, we have a duty to do our best to solve the problems people have with accessing information, thus improving their ability to make better decisions. Especially when you have someone as close as your parents involved in the struggle of that kind of medical decision-making process, this brings your research closer to "home".

2   Health Informatics

Some medical professionals I observed could have spent more time caring for people. Instead, I observed them struggling with poorly designed technology. I started thinking about how I could improve these processes. You know, I could have done my research in many other areas, but I gradually moved into health-related research, and I stayed there for most of my career since.

   Over the years I have often contemplated on my research. I would question myself if I should do more research in health? In the early 2000's a colleague of mine invited me to join a team that was working on the proposal for an Australian Research Council grant to collaborate with a Breast Cancer Advocacy Group. I met with her and her friend and colleague that was a breast cancer "survivor" who was one of the lead people in that Breast Cancer Group Advocacy. She spoke in great detail to us about the problems women with breast cancer were having in finding relevant information while they were faced with this disease. As a result of that conversation and fit with my desire to assist we offered to partner with them to work on an online system to help them meet their information needs. Effectively the research aimed at creating an online intelligent portal that would allow for better communication and better information provision for women with breast cancer and their carers. In essence taking a comprehensive, whole family approach to support and to provide suitable, quality information for everybody about breast cancer. I was kind of very "ripe" to healthcare-based research by then, as I was struggling myself to find suitable information about my father's condition. I knew that ways of finding the right medical information needed to be improved back then and I think it's still a problem. My overall hope was that maybe with smart tools will get people better equipped and informed with what information they needed to make better healthcare decisions. With that Breast Cancer Knowledge Online portal that we proposed and developed we demonstrated how it can be done. I was one of the architects for this system contributing on the technical side of this research (Burstein et al. 2005).

   I led the development of the Breast Cancer Knowledge Online portal initiative, funded by a series of research grants over 15 years. The aim of BCKOnline was to empower the individual user by determining the type of information which will best suit her needs at any point in time throughout the cancer trajectory. The BCKOnline portal presented users with a data from other public resources carefully curated by breast cancer survivors and other well informed domain experts. The initiative received many accolades and awards (https://rcblog.erc.monash.edu.au/blog/2021/09/breast-cancer-knowledge-online/).

   For the past 20 years, it's still the case that government is pouring a lot of resources into creating various special information sources for carers, for patients, for families, for you name it. But people still prefer *"Dr Google"*. The truth is that people still use *Dr Google* and *Professor Wikipedia* when they need information about medical conditions. Sadly, health informatics literacy has not being promoted enough, so people do not know how to get access to high quality information they need in a form they can sufficiently understand. I still think that, probably coming from my own experience. I wish I knew more about certain medical conditions and about the kind of medications that doctors were prescribing for these conditions. Theoretically, health care for patients is as good as it can be. In practice, we're often facing a very patriarchal, hierarchical sort of approach to healthcare. You could also say "matriarchal" because there are women doctors as well. It mostly takes a "we know better what is good for you" approach to patients' treatment. However, the patients, and carers still hope for more of an egalitarian system. This what a patient-centred care should be about.

You can provide a person with information to give them the opportunity to make a decision, but they should be educated enough to make sense of it. You need to be informing them about their own condition and teaching them about what's feasible, and what's not; I think this is something that could be done much better. And you know this new generation that is walking around with their smartphones and having access to all new technologies which are quick and good at finding information, but nobody's teaching them how to evaluate its quality or how to use it best within their context. I know at school, they are now taught that, don't use Wikipedia, but that's not true either, because Wikipedia is not the worst resource. If you ask me, social media is used far too often and it can be really bad. Much worse than Google or Wikipedia. With no expert control on the quality of the social medial information - there is no way to check the advice you can get from these networks.

Grant: Exactly. Frada, I would have to agree. Much worse. I often describe the WWW not as the World Wide Web, but as the World Wild Web.

Frada: Glad we agree. I'm talking from my own experience as a patient, a carer and also as a researcher. It effectively means that for the past 20 years all projects I've been involved in are done in a digital healthcare context. So, they're all in some sort of health informatics and human-centered health information systems. I have supervised maybe 30-plus research students during these years and all those projects were health informatics related. For example, we looked at the way people use social media to support information seeking sustainability and how it factored into resilience. Especially for people facing chronic conditions. It's been very interesting actually. There is a lot of room of improvement. But I don't know whether the findings from researchers are finding their ways to a full implementation as easily as possible. There is a lot of excitement in many areas of health informatics and people are looking at many technical innovations within digital health. I have heard people say the same about agriculture and the same about manufacturing maybe. However, in healthcare the questions are often about life and death, or at least reducing the mental pressure because you feel like you are walking in the dark about your condition—seems like a worthy cause to invest future efforts in.

You simply do not get smart enough interfaces to give you the best, most relevant and quality information. You could make a better decision based on the information provided to you. Like I told you, my research training is in decision support since I was in my 20s, so I've done enough research and believe I have enough background expertise to tell you that if you look at good theory of decision-making it provides a lot of useful learnings which could be adopted in developing more effective health information systems. Theories grounded in cognitive psychology and other behavioural sciencies that researchers have full access to and appreciation for. All these together with better health literacy could do much more for digital healthcare and for patients' wellbeing.

But today there is a huge knowledge gap. When you look at the smart young doctors, they are pretty technically savvy: if they need an App or need clinical decision support. They think they can do it all by themselves and without any expert ICT research help, it's hilarious.

You know it took me a while to even feel appreciated as an expert when I talk to doctors. I will never forget a project—I went with my Post Doc to a hospital and a resident professor was so skeptical about us being there. I simply could not convince him that, we have extra value to bring by establishing a research collaboration. He was totally dismissive of anything to do with IT research. Very often, the clinicians see the technology they have in place as given, but don't have much interest in reflecting if it can be improved and how. Or maybe, they were just too busy with clinical pressure at the time? I would say that not every medical professor is like that, but that one was totally dismissive. I was so upset. I just basically walked out of that research proposal but, I believed that things could've been done better, but this depends on how digital health is taught to medical students. Since then I came across a different experience while conducting research in multiple hospitals and the findings were mutually enlightening.

3   Multidisciplinary Research

I have put my heart and soul into trying to establish connections with the medical faculty at my current university and we've developed digital health courses for them. But the challenge is that IT academics and the medical profession speak different languages. We have a huge gap between us. We talk about multidisciplinary nature of research and it's very hard to achieve actually. It's not simple. I've been doing it because it's fun and you learn so much from the other partners. But it requires a lot of effort. It requires that you open up and admit that you have this boundary in your expertise. And, to having a high respect for the other party. Then somehow, you define a problem to address with your research that you "own" together.

But you know Grant, that I mentioned to you that Breast Cancer Knowledge Online project and what came out of it at the end was not just that portal that we developed. What truly came out of it was an architecture that has been rolled in multiple disciplines. For example, Heart Health Online which we also built on the same principles. We have also done a project with medical colleagues from Deakin University to help patients with provision of information on stress and depression. So, the same architectural approach was taken in all these projects. Importantly what came out of these projects was also a research methodology that we called "inclusive research" design [see as described by my colleagues and me in McKemmish et al. 2012]. It's based on "value sensitive" design. I don't know whether you've heard about "value sensitive" design. It is defined as the unity of three dimensions—conceptual, technical, and empirical (Friedman et al. 2002)

Grant: No, sorry Frada

Frada: Actually, it's not only applied to IT systems, but it can also be applied to any design where the values and needs of the users aimed to be considered explicitly and dynamically as they change. It's about treating future users as equal participants of your research, and giving them a voice and space for having their values explicitly expressed and embedded into what you propose to design. The challenge for the ICT researchers is to clearly define the Conceptual model which could drive this innovation. The collaborators from medical and other disciplines are mostly interested in Empirical and Technical outcomes. However, without the conceptual clarity behind the innovative model—there is no way to produce publishable research contributions.

This is actually a very important principle for collaborative health informatics research. A lot of researchers working in other applied areas conduct project by project almost like an academic "assembly line". Each project has a defined start and it has a defined finish. When you do research in digital health, however, and if you do a good job, you quite often finish up with developing such a close relationship with your medical partners they feel like they want to go on and do more research with you. This is because they realize that there is so much more for them to do, and they have much more access to funding compared to us as ICT academics by the way. But that means that their needs change as research progresses. They change dynamically—so you need to re-define your research into a new cycle. If you let the research direction to be driven by medical research collaborators you will come up with some sort of artifacts meeting their requirements to an extent, but they're not good enough to be published in our high-quality academic outlets. What I'm really talking about here is again the disconnect between different expectations in our fields of research and practice. For example, the first project we did to design a BCKOnline portal we used the top of the range technology and we got access to it for academic purposes. We developed an initial prototype which was good enough in academic terms, and we could publish about it. It was funded by the Australian Research Council project, so the Department of Health was involved, and the Breast Cancer Advocacy community group was involved. The Department of Health gave us money and then they moved on. They were not interested in maintaining what we proposed. The community group had no money to take it over, but they really liked the concept, and they wanted us to continue developing the information resource and make it available for their members. We had the platform installed on our server and it started being used and people started to publicize it among women. This meant that we had to look for some continuous funding to keep the portal alive so that the women and families who were interested in accessing a quality curated portal content with the carefully selected and classified resources could still get access to it.

At times, my other colleagues said, "you know, the project's over."

My response was "Yes, I know, but can we stop the community served with these resources? We should be able to do something for them while they need our help".

But the project funding was over, so how could we look after it continuously into the future and maintain it? I tried to explain this to the Community group that got a taste of what the innovation was, and they saw value in it. You could not easily explain to them that now it's all over and thank you very much. Goodbye. For myself to be honest it could not have worked that way. So, I found a few groups of students to redevelop the platform from scratch. Because for the community group the technical innovation was not the main crux of what they wanted the resource to do, and so we moved to an open-source solution.

We formulated a task for a group of students as part of their Industrial Experience Project. These students redeveloped our portal as a smart database using an open-source software. To populate this "smart database we still needed a deep expertise of those women from the Breast Cancer community group to create and select the appropriate resources and it became more of what I would call a smart knowledge repository. It had to be indexed in a particular way and the students brought in very advanced search engine that was open-source that we could use for free. It was called Lucene™ and then eventually re-designed it using Apache Solr search platform You could just attach it to any SQL database, but it was doing very smart indexing and allowed us to implement a faceted search for appropriate resources. So, with students help and new technologies we developed the second prototype, and it was just basic technically, but it was created by students—so everybody had a chance to learn and we kept the portal "alive."

But prototype revisions required continuous research thinking. What are the possibilities? Where is the value adding capabilities of using technology rather than focusing on what you know. At the end of the project, we finished with a good demonstrator for what can be done, but it's very old fashioned now. Not many solid technical publications came out of it, but we achieved something for the community group and for the greater good. We had the methodology paper which came out of it that I mentioned earlier, and it was fun to write. I was lucky by that time I was already an Associate Professor. So, for me it wasn't a big deal how many more publications I have, but I always give it as an example for younger researchers. They have to be much more strategic when they are conducting applied IT research. If you approach your research strategically - you can achieve a "win-win" situation - to meet your collaborators' expectations, while also generating sufficient theoretical innovation to advance knowledge in your discipline and produce quality publications as is expected from our academic roles.

So, when I moved to the other projects, I was very proud of what we've done in BCKOnline space. Then Andrew (Stranieri) liked what we had done, and we started to collaborate more looking into smart information portals in general. Having a solid prototype already developed and tested allowed a lot of little future projects to be attached to it. It was a unique experience for me, but that was not a driver. The driver is always looking at the excited eyes of the participants and hearing about how we had empowered them to make better decisions concerning their health and the health of their loved ones. Also, for example, there were examples of a breast cancer nurse that was recommending our portal to her patients and also a surgeon who mentioned our portal as a source of trust worthy information for his patient recommendations. The alternative is still - "Dr Google".

Often, when I am looking for health information specifically, my heart bleeds. Governments promote health databases. But I don't know who they tested them with. I've been observing how they seem to ignore the personalization part of these on-line resources. They keep creating these new generic systems, but one size doesn't fit all. What we learned first from talking to that community is that it's not just about demographics or age. Information portals need to tailor language, content and approach at a personal health literacy level and life context. For example, if you are a young unmarried lady just being diagnosed with breast cancer then you should be presented with a list of questions and options suited to your life circumstance. These would be different when compared to a grandmother who had children and grandchildren, or if you have young family. So, you look for much more tailored information needs about the similar health conditions, but with different personal circumstances driving the information requirements.

Doctors appreciate the approach, but they're so busy themselves to give truely personalized assistance. So, if you were a patient then they would give you paper-based pamphlets or they can send you to a generic website. Generic websites are often too shallow in content so you may find little by way of information you are after, or get scared by the amount of technical details it contains. I have spoken to research participants who have said that when they were diagnosed with breast cancer they did not want to be immediately exposed to reading about palliative care. If you start exploring your options based generic search you can be overwhelmed by an "avalanche" of information. This is actually a term we heard from our research participants. You get bogged down in the information that may be irrelevant, or hard to interpret to start with, but this is when it's critical to know what your options are and why should you choose one or the other.

It's exactly what I experienced with my father because, you know, the doctors kept pouring information at me and they were focused on worst-case scenarios. For example, a few months after his accident I was asked if I had arranged the wheelchair? I said, what are you telling me? Is he not going to walk anymore? This approach made me feel very dis-empowered and you are assumed to know everything that is happening and why. It feels like the more educated you look and sound then doctors assume that you know or understand more complex terminology and the details of the conditions. But for most people they do not have the ability to instantly comprehend complex medical issues.

Grant: In terms of "value centered "design, how is that different to "user centered design" in which the users are involved in product design and development? This design methodology is often taught in IT courses.

Frada: It's completely different. User centered design is a very interesting concept if you look at how it's been prescribed. It is included within the International Organization for Standardization (ISO) standards focused on "human-centered design". Basically, user centered design step by step can be defined as: consult the user to start with and then iteratively evaluate your prototype with the user. It's all driven by user requirements. The users you are consulting are meant to be able to tell you up front what their requirements are. You have worked in the IT industry long enough to know that no user in their good mind will know upfront what they truly need and require in detail. I have had users tell me that they don't know what they want, but if I could show them what could be done, then they would tell me whether the solution fits their needs. Also, to be honest it is quite often about expectations. It's not about what they need. It is like looking at our financial systems. That's the best example. They give us everything we need, don't they? But ask me if they are user friendly, or designed in a user centered way? That's a different story. They can be hard to use by people who have not accessed computers as much as we have. I've been educated about computers and systems my whole life, and if I can't quite comprehend the on-line financial system then I can guarantee that people 10–15 years older than me will also have problems. I feel for them. But even the younger generation, who are much more technologically intuitive, can often have problems using on-line systems. You need people to explain to you the values they will put into the system you plan to develop for them and also their needs. I mentioned earlier that decision we made about using open source software, for example, for the BCKOnline portal infrastructure as opposed to the top of the range technology. Of course, if we had used top of the range technology, we could have achieved probably better technical results, but the users did not care. They were not concerned at all with what happens in the back-end of our system. All they needed was an effective and particular online search interface delivering information suitable to their circumstances. Their needs from the system will differ individually from the first point of use through to the final point of use. Each person's journey through treatment and support could be different. I do not think that user centered design assumes that user requirements will change over time. I have supervised a whole PhD project about user expectations where we found that user expectations are different to user requirements. They are also mentioned as part of user centered design, but nobody tells you how to acquire them. The outcome of the project was a whole list of questions that the designers could put into their requirements engineering phase to elicit expectations, not just requirements.

Grant: Frada, earlier you spoke about I guess the "gap" that exists between researchers and the doctors, or you know, we could even say more broadly between academia and industry. How do you see us bridging that gap more successfully into the future?

Frada: With great difficulty, I must say.

Grant: Or is there a need to bridge the gap?

Frada: Absolutely. I think every researcher needs to ask themselves this question earlier rather than later. If you are driven by pure career advancements in academia, you probably do not feel very concerned about the relevance of your research to industry. If you look at scientific research in technologies, for example AI, which is becoming more and more popular nowadays - this question can not be avoided any more. We were working with AI technologies in the 1990s and we knew what the problems were occuring when people offered such technologies as expert systems, for example, for real-world implementation and embracement. The same problems exist now, but the popularity of AI is growing because for a while it was driven by technologists and people stopped thinking about the lessons we learned from developing expert systems in the 90s. Because there were no answers found to those problems then, and they are catching up with answers now For example, who should be responsible for the errors made by the medical system with AI at its core? The researchers have to offer some answers to such questions to gain more trust when it comes to offering industry-level solutions. I am glad to see that there are serious advancements offered by way of regulating how much of technology "black box" can be embedded into the healthcare systems and what ethical considerations should be observed (if not followed directly). Lately I have been doing presentations about industry-led and industry-based research. The existence of research driven organizations like Cooperative Research Centres (CRC) Programs demonstrate that new ideas can attract a huge amount of money that industry and government invest into such initiatives. It is driven by industry needs. They want researchers to come together to address their needs. We join together in project teams as researchers and they define the problem for us. In return they expect that we give them results and then they appropriate the results and off they go. There is an expectation that it will be kind of a fair share of results in some way. But the issues of shared IP and legal risk management is looked after at the CRC level. That's a different and complicated story.

The process of producing high quality publications based on the results of industry-led research it is very challenging at least in my discipline. Because you know it takes 2 years to get publication out in the information system field. No industry partner would be interested to stay in that project for so long and help with all the revisions and submissions. Hence, as I said earlier, if you are an early career researcher, and need publications for advancing your positions - industry-led research can take a lot of time and effort with no guarantee of publishing the results.

On the other hand, I have supervised so many research students and all of them have been doing bits and pieces of research with industry collaborators in what I call "industry-based research" settings. In this case, the researchers define the research problem we aim to address. We more or less have very solid conceptual theoretical understanding of what we try to research, but we need the context. This is the context that industry partners could provide to us if the ideas are relevant to their needs. Having all these connections within healthcare institutions was very fortunate to me and my students. Over time I developed long-term collaborations with doctors and other health professionals. They often get very excited if a research student presents an idea to them and they often have light-bulb moments. They suddenly understand how research could assist their dataset analysis, for example. But it is not their life-blood research and they're not dependent on any risks if a student project does not lead to any useful results. It's a kind of a "true" research, take it, or leave it. The impact needs to be very clear, if they don't like it they will tell you. You cannot go into such projects with high expectations on the level of practical implementation which will follow from the outcomes produced by researchers. That's what I tried to explain to my students. I know how hospitals work, and they simply don't have the extra time to deploy the system and they always have a shortage of IT staff.

Another thing is that there are certain ways things are done in the hospital and in the medical domain in general that they're not going to change for you overnight. There are some constraints and traditions there that you're working within. Sometimes they do not like the system that they are working with, but if you tell them that they need to redevelop it completely because of your research results they might say, "Seriously, we just invested lots of money to implement it and it is what it is."

Healthcare institutions and services experience a huge need for improvement of their IT infrastructure. So, I feel like if I can help a little bit, if my PhD students can help a little bit also, then I am happy to invest my knowledge and energy to collaborate with them in a meaningful way. For example, at the moment, I have two projects which are looking at the cognitive biases and the use of seminal decision-making theories to underpin the design of medical alerts and reminders for doctors to make better decisions in, for example, prescribing medications and pathology tests. Will the outcomes be implemented practically? Probably not immediately, but at least we've done our duty. We've demonstrated to the doctors what is wrong with the ways these processes are done currently and we've done it by conducting a very good, rigorous research. In turn I am confident that my students will get their PhDs and gain a lot of very valuable experience from these collaborations. They could have done PhD in other areas, but I think my duty is to try something for those doctors who otherwise may not be able to recognize the opportunities our research can offer.

Grant: I think it's interesting Frada, I talked about my work to students sometimes and I put up an example of a grant I got in the past. It was for about $25,000, small money in comparison to other grants. But from that I then I built a platform which goes online and with thousands of people registered. Helping people to practise their speech and social skills. I explain to the students that it is free and then the feedback came from one single user. In basic terms the feedback thanks me for the platform and how it has changed their lives. I then explain to students that this single paragraph is worth more than $25,000, even though I never heard from this user again.

Frada: Such a good example and thank you for sharing.

Grant: Thank you for contributing to this book, Frada. For agreeing to be interviewed for this chapter and for telling a part of your story. One last question. What do you hope to get out of this contribution personally?

Frada: Look, I'm at the point of my career where one more publication doesn't really matter. Saying this, I think, the benefits are for me to reflect on my research journey. It was very useful for me explaining myself and explaining to myself what I've done and how I've done it, and why I've done it the way I did. This is probably the opportunity I would appreciate most - because of our interview for the book. I wonder if there will be any opportunity for feedback from the readers. That kind of exposure can be scary for me even to think about at times. I don't know how useful my story and opinions will be for the readers, but it's going to be in the public domain and obviously very personal. For me contributing to this book is like a mentoring exercise. I wanted to tell the real story about doing research in digital health the way I did it, the way I approached it, let it be right or wrong. I believe that I deserve to talk about it after 20 years of having done something. It's more like a "lessons learned" rather than a "how to" story, I suppose.

Grant: Thank you so much Frada for your deep and personal story.

References

Burstein F, Fisher J, McKemmish S, Manaszewicz R, Malhotra P. User centred quality health information provision: benefits and challenges. In: Proceedings of the 38th Annual Hawaii International Conference on System Sciences. IEEE: Piscataway; 2005. p. 138c. https://ieeexplore.ieee.org/abstract/document/1385515.

Friedman B, Kahn P, Borning A. Value sensitive design: theory and methods. Univ Washington Tech Rep. 2002;2:12.

McKemmish S, Burstein F, Manaszewicz R, Fisher J, Evans J. Inclusive research design: unravelling the double hermeneutic spiral. Inf Commun Soc. 2012;15(7):1106–35.

Better Health Through Integrative Medicine: A Pursuit of Lived Experience

Peter De Lorenzo and Sitalakshmi Venkatraman

Abstract Integrative medicine (IM) refers to the medical practice that aims for a balance in using evidence-based conventional medicine with complementary and alternative medicine (CAM), or therapy interventions having a holistic view on individual health and well-being. Despite IM emergence in Australia, its contribution to the quality of healthcare from the perspectives of medical practitioners, pharmacists, consumers and other stakeholders is not well understood. In this chapter, we describe our pursuit of lived experience as individuals embracing IM with a shared goal and as IT professionals towards providing a better information awareness to the wider community.

Peter De Lorenzo, the CEO of UnityHealth Pty Ltd (www.unityhealth.com.au), the founding owner of IMgateway.net, through his lived experience shares his successful lifestyle transition that has paved the way for establishing meaningful connections through this evidence-based online digital platform. Peter's suffering from chronic eczema for the first 40 years of his life had raised his awareness of IM and passion for pain relief and improved health for himself, his family and the community.

Sitalakshmi Venkatraman (Sita), Discipline Leader of Business Analytics in Melbourne Polytechnic describes her lived experience from being raised in a family embracing Ayurvedic Medicine and becoming a passionate IT educator and Health Informatics researcher. Sita describes her personal and career journey towards developing her research interest in the effective use of IT for a positive impact on the patient community.

Peter and Sita, with their expertise in new generation digital services, together collaborate with the belief that the continued journey of IMgateway facilitates a pathway of health and understanding of a person's life, termed as 'holistic'. Through this chapter, we aspire to promote this holistic approach to healthcare as it imbibes

P. De Lorenzo (✉)
UnityHealth, Kew, VIC, Australia
e-mail: peter.delorenzo@unityhealth.com.au

S. Venkatraman
Melbourne Polytechnic, Preston, VIC, Australia

A. Stranieri et al. (eds.), *Research Partners with Lived Experience*,
https://doi.org/10.1007/978-981-97-0033-2_8

103

evidence-based preventative health principles of safety, efficacy and applicability. Based on the personal experiences, we find a massive need in our community for bridging the gaps witnessed with the integration of conventional and complementary medicine and providing better health for the wider community.

Keywords Integrative medicine (IM) · Complementary and alternative medicine (CAM) · Adverse drug reaction (ADR) · Digital education

1 Our Journey

Peter's narrative:

> I am immensely grateful for my lived experience I was subject to from my birth in 1959 and throughout my childhood, youth, adulthood, fatherhood and as a businessman. All my lived experience centred around my health and wellness. I learned consciously and sub-consciously through my lived experiences with many others, my quiet reflections and some critical thinking. I suffered from eczema as an infant which became chronic for the first 40 years of my life. With my mother's support, I visited numerous healthcare professionals and received various treatments and products with limited or no success. My mother relentlessly researched healthcare books, articles and medical journals, in order to help my condition. My mother's quest was no doubt instrumental in raising my awareness and passion for pain relief and improved health.
>
> From a teenager, exposed to the suffering of my young grandmother, to an intermittent carer for my mother and my sister (all of whom died from cancer); I faced challenging and confronting experiences over the decades. This no doubt fed my purpose. This purpose was fueled by a Complementary and Alternative Medicine (CAM) approach to health and witnessing improved quality of life and prolonged time with family. These experiences were immeasurably valuable in raising my awareness of a patient-centred approach to health and healing.
>
> After successfully establishing a career in Information Technology and large corporate businesses, I made the decision to form my own healthcare company, UnityHealth, www.unityhealth.com.au, at the age of 40.
>
> The last 20 plus years working in the business has been the bedrock for my personal growth in actively collaborating, exchanging and befriending some remarkable professionals across the spectrum of academia, research, medicine, pharmacy, community, allied healthcare and students.
>
> A more recent enlightenment was the positive lived experience I received as a carer for my father. Through a changed diet, improved lifestyle, improved sleep and CAM support from an integrative doctor; my father was able to reverse his diabetes, hypertension and dementia in his eighties and eliminate all his medications. After an amazing life, my father died in December 2022, just short of his 91st birthday.

Sita's narrative:

> During my childhood days, I was always trying to overcome my health issues due to my weak constitution. I was suffering from tonsilitis very often and nervousness. However, due to my family tradition of holistic health belief in Ayurvedic Medicine, I was able to recover from the majority of my health issues with CAM. I was raised in an environment witnessing my grandfather and father adopting this holistic approach to health. My grandfather was able to treat his diabetes with self-motivated home tests and Ayurvedic remedies. He lived

an active life even at the age of 89 years. I strongly believe that he would have lived the full 120 years as per Ayurveda's healthy life expectancy but for a road accident. My father, who is 92 years old, practices yoga regularly and with the help of Ayurvedic principles and remedies, adopts self-care without resorting to conventional medicine as much as possible.

Raised in such an environment, I had little knowledge about conventional medicines until my marriage. It was while taking care of my mother-in-law who was suffering from a variety of health issues such as, Irritable Bowel Syndrome (IBS), anxiety and headaches as well as osteoporosis, I had the privilege of gaining much knowledge about conventional medicines and their interactions with our body and mind. The medications prescribed for one issue invariably had adverse reactions with the other. My husband and I being in the education profession, the clinic she visited was within our university campus and it housed a variety of specialists and CAM practitioners. We were fortunate that a holistic approach including Homeopathic treatments at the clinic provided her with a more personalised remedy. She could survive successfully for 20 more years with a combination of conventional and CAM treatments.

My lived experience of witnessing the health journeys undertaken by my family members have shaped my beliefs towards accepting other forms of treatments such as Homeopathy. Personally, by adopting a holistic approach I have overcome my own health issues which included a severe sciatic attack. I believe that each method of healing practices in Ayurveda, Homeopathy, TCM, naturopathy, etc. that can complement conventional medicine has its own set of advantages and disadvantages and the impact would vary from one person to another. Hence, an awareness of these principles would be very useful for an individual to arrive at how a combination of these treatments could be undertaken, safely minimising any adverse side-effects while maximising the positive impact. In my opinion such an awareness of IM would aid in building a therapeutic doctor-patient relationship for achieving positive results through a quicker recovery process. It would foster an open communication between patients and doctors with a shared partnership for enhancing patient wellbeing.

In recent years, health promotion and individual-based interventions for disease prevention are given importance worldwide for minimising the burden of diseases and associated risk factors. It has taken my lived experience of several decades to gain sufficient knowledge and IM awareness for embracing a more preventive and holistic healthcare. However, I strongly feel that the recent advances in digital technologies could be leveraged effectively to empower everyone in the community by providing more control over one's health and wellbeing.

My personal health journey has paved the way for transforming my research interests from a pure IT discipline to an interdisciplinary health informatics domain with a focus on CAM and IM awareness for the benefit of the society. In Australia, for nearly 15 years in the past, my research focus in Health Informatics started to take some meaningful contribution while working with the Health Informatics Research Group under the leadership of Dr. Andrew Stranieri. Furthermore, about a decade ago when I witnessed UnityHealth winning the Australian innovation award for health category, I was motivated very much to collaborate with UnityHealth's research pursuits in this direction. I learnt more about IM and adverse drug reactions through Peter and his team. I was able to channel some of my student capstone projects in developing meaningful outcomes.

Though our initial lived experience were quite different, we share a common goal of developing an innovative new generation digital service to facilitate a pathway of holistic health through the understanding of a person's life. Our journey in the past decade has overlapping research interests (De Lorenzo 2007; Venkatraman and Stranieri 2012; O'Brien et al. 2020). UnityHealth's IMgateway (https://www.imgateway.net), a key system launched in 2001, aims to bridge the gap in the integration of conventional and complementary medicine. The purpose of this chapter is to share our collaborative journey of enhancing Imgateway to promote information awareness of IM and ADR to a variety of stakeholders in the community. The challenges of ADRs described in the next section form the compelling reason for the development of projects in our collaborative research journey.

2   The Challenges of ADRs

Our literature reviews concur with each of our lived experience that CAM forms a wide range of healthcare medicines and therapies that can be adopted for specific health conditions or health benefits to suit each one's requirements (De Lorenzo 2007; Venkatraman and Stranieri 2012; O'Brien et al. 2020). In the past decade, there has been an increased uptake of CAM by consumers who are embracing many forms and models of health to take control of their own well-being. This trend is also attributed to CAM being considered around the world as accessible, affordable and culturally acceptable within their healthcare options (BMA British Medical Association 1993; Australian Institute of Health and Welfare 2020; Ng 2020). According to the World Health Organisation, 80% of the world's population and 70% of the Australian community use some form of traditional or complementary medicine (World Health Organization 2022). Until now, there has not been an easy, evidence-based way for the consumer to identify the likelihood of an adverse interaction between their medicines and particular herbs, supplements or food. Research studies show that 50% of Australians who report using complementary and alternative medicines, are concurrently using conventional medicines (Gallego et al. 2019; Steel et al. 2018). Yet, a high per cent do not report their use of complementary medicines to their doctor. The number of people integrating their treatment regimen is still rising with an increase in complementary medicine expenditure.

In Australia, more than 300 million prescriptions for medications are dispensed every year, including 90% of older Australians receiving at least one prescription in the last 12 months. Almost one in two Australians report taking a medicine in any 2-week period (Australian Institute of Health and Welfare 2020; Australian Bureau of Statistics 2020). The estimated cost of medicines to Australians accounts for approximately 12% of annual healthcare expenditure, including both prescription and over-the-counter medicines (Australian Institute of Health and Welfare 2020). The high frequency of medication results in medication-related problems that include adverse medicine events, adverse medicine reactions, inappropriate medicine selection, under- or overdosing, medication use without an indication, medicine–medicine interactions and untreated indications (Strand et al. 1990). Adverse medicine reaction also termed as an adverse drug reaction is a subset of adverse medicine events, where the harm is directly caused by administration of a medication (Edwards and Aronson 2000).

In Australia, a comprehensive home medication review reports that one in five people were identified as suffering an adverse medication event, at the time of the review (Easton et al. 2009). Overall, research reports published over the last 2 decades consistently show that, with an increase in CAM uptake, addressing ADRs to support medication safety is a major challenge to the Australian healthcare system (Easton et al. 2009; Schmid et al. 2022).

CAM and natural therapies contribute to 70% of Australian uptake and remains consistently high over time. While the Australian complementary medicine industry reached $5.2 billion in revenues in 2018 and is providing a significant contribution to the economy, there are serious concerns in the standardised death rate due to ADRs increasing from 4.9 in 2020 to 5.1 deaths in 2021 (Easton et al. 2009; Schmid et al. 2022). In a recent study, 56% of patients suffered from a previous history of an ADR, and for about 50% of cases, the cause was due to multiple medicines (PSA Pharmaceutical Society of Australia 2019). While 87% cases were considered preventable, 13% of patients were still readmitted due to an ADR within the 12 months indicating the lack of support services and reliable information. Hence, medication-related hospital admissions represent a serious health issue and are associated with significant costs to the Australian healthcare system. Australian hospitals report greater injuries and health costs due to ADRs indicating a requirement of considerable urgency for IM literacy.

In Australia, more than 17% of general hospital admissions and 30% of admissions in the elderly population are the result of ADRs (Schmid et al. 2022). The cost of ADRs are more than 15% of the total expenditure on direct hospital costs. In addition, the burden of ADRs on the Australian healthcare system is high, and account for considerable morbidity and mortality which increases markedly each year. Reduction of loss of life and costs that are attributable to ADR avoidance is an urgent requirement. This has been the focus of our research investigations for more than a decade. The Commonwealth Government of Australia has been supporting only a basic level of information with respect to complementary medicines through a not-for-profit internet-based advisory service (MedicineWise). Though established in 1998, the online service still lacks support for ADR avoidance and lacks rigorous links to the underlying science and evidence-based (Australian Commission on Safety and Quality in Health Care 2020). This formed the key motivation for UnityHealth to provide the required support services in the domain of IM. Based on the personal experiences, we find a massive need in our community for bridging the gaps witnessed with the integration of conventional and complementary medicine.

Peter's narrative:

If quality and up-to-date information on the pharmacology, pharmacokinetics and most importantly clinical efficacy and safety profile of CAM are available to healthcare professionals, they can confidently advise their patients (who are often taking multiple drugs). Availability of the same evidenced-based information for patients that prompts them to liaise with their healthcare professional will greatly improve the practitioner-patient therapeutic relationship.

Key IM support services, including pioneering initiatives such as IMgateway.net and a QACPD accredited education programme for doctors, led by Professor Avni Sali, were the first of their kind established more than two decades ago. These, together with fruitful partnerships with university researchers, qualified healthcare professionals and Australia's healthcare organisations, are helping Australia lead other countries in healthcare industry education and training.

UnityHealth developed and enhanced several systems including a database called IMgateway to provide instant alerts on how a prescribed drug interacts with complementary medicines and foods, and an educational website called iTherapeutics. In 2013, two of UnityHealth's systems were recognised and awarded for Innovation and subsequently represented Australian Innovation in Hong Kong in late 2013. UnityHealth's iTherapeutics training programme, which is used by over 90% of Australian pharmacies, was awarded the Education prize at the Victorian iAwards. The IMgateway database of UnityHealth won a National Award in the Health category.

Australia now has a better trained pharmacy and healthcare workforce with access to consistent and structured online educational programmes that are helping them know what questions to ask of their customers and clients and make informed recommendations. It is gratifying to offer this training equally in regional and rural areas. Further, the greatest satisfaction comes from the impact the training and information databases can have on the end consumer who receives more current, high-quality information, improved advice from both the healthcare professional as well as pharmacy staff. A high percentage of complementary medicines are purchased in pharmacy by Australians. However, our research studies continue to evaluate the systems and information databases used by healthcare professionals and consumers and how they meet the IM stakeholder needs'.

3   Meeting IM Stakeholder Needs

The growth of complementary medicine poses a range of dilemmas for IM stakeholders such as healthcare professionals and consumers or CAM users. It is becoming increasingly more necessary for doctors to be educated in IM, otherwise their patients will go elsewhere. There is a need for doctors to have a common understanding of CAM treatments undertaken by the majority of their patients. Doctors who are familiar with evidence-based complementary medicine modalities can be regarded as more completely educated in general medicine and are more likely to discuss complementary medicine options with their patients in a non-judgmental way (Ung et al. 2018). In Australia, it is reported that more members of the public visit a complementary medicine health professional than a doctor (von Conrady and Bonney 2017).

Peter's working experience with the Australasian Integrative Medicine Association (www.AIMA.net.au) and learnings from various member doctors highlighted the urgent need for the medical professional to have access to CAM education training. According to Peter, 'The 7-minute mainstream doctor's appointment never satisfactorily served my needs for a preventative, holistic-based intervention, not purely based on a symptom driven recommendation'.

Today's healthcare professionals can no longer ignore the rising interest in complementary medicine by the public (CMA Complementary Medicines Australia 2022; Huang et al. 2019). There is an enormous opportunity for doctors to expand their services by offering scientifically validated complementary medicine modalities in their treatment armamentarium (Australian Institute of Health and Welfare 2018a; Commonwealth of Australia 2019). Doctors will be better able to serve their patients by integrating the science of conventional medicine with the science of complementary medicine (Ng et al. 2020). To meet the needs of healthcare professionals, the IMgateway database was enhanced by developing case scenarios along with rich coverage of monographs and branded location-based drug information tailored to international regions through the established collaboration with MIMS. Figure 1 shows an example of an interactions check the healthcare professionals could make using IMgateway for supporting an evidence-based and informed CAM consultation with their patients.

While the clinical data was made readily available to clinicians through IMgateway, the rise in self care created a need for similar, evidence-based information about potential interactions, to be available to Consumers. Through our own personal health journeys, we have witnessed the effective use of CAM amongst our own family members dealing with certain health issues. According to Sitalakshmi Venkatraman, 'the advancements in IT could be leveraged in providing evidence-based information on CAM for the empowerment of each individual to make an

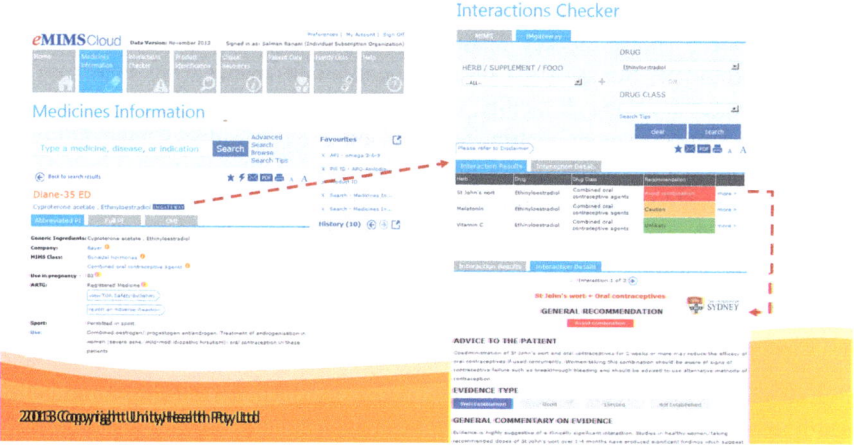

Fig. 1 IMgateway supporting interactions check during a CAM consultation

informed decision about their own health and wellbeing and more importantly to benefit the wider CAM consumer community'.

The IMgateway interactions database was subsequently trailed and assessed for consumer use through the energy and inspiration of Sally Percival Wood, supported by Tricia Greenway, a consumer engagement adviser for this consumer led, co-designed project.

In order to test out its usability, a research project was established and managed by Associate Professor Kylie O'Brien to seek feedback on how its design could be improved, and to assess its potential usefulness as a consumer resource (O'Brien et al. 2020; Greenstock et al. 2013). A secondary aim was to investigate attitudes and behaviour with respect to CAM use. CAM therapies support mind-body interventions that combine many methods such as meditation to enhance the mind's positive effects on the body. Since CAM use is often high in cancer patients, the survey was circulated among members of the Review and Survey Group of the Breast Cancer Network of Australia (BCNA). Participants then answered questions about their experience using the IMgateway database including the ease of use and the nature of its features or valuable improvements for a consumer. All feedback provided was examined independently and the results were published in the European Journal of Integrative Medicine (O'Brien et al. 2020). The BCNA consumer group's inputs gained through the study complement the functional requirements that have been derived from the experience of 43,000 doctors, pharmacists and allied health care professionals and education of more than 90 percent of pharmacists since 2001. The key findings of the research led to the development of a Consumer App prototype aiding the potential value of the IMgateway database to consumer decision-making behaviour in relation to CAM use. Figure 2 shows the consumer-led research project meetings that were supported by IM stakeholders—BCNA members and others.

A group of students from a tertiary institution developed the first prototype of the IMgateway Consumer App as a Capstone Project under the guidance of the second author. Figure 3 shows the key features of IMgateway App developed as a co-designed prototype. Some of the improvements made in the App, such as user-friendly navigation, a search facility, saving prescriptions and medicine reminders for patients, were consumer-centric and in response to the feedback gained through the research project. Further improvements were made to the next prototype development of the IMgateway Consumer App. Advanced search with auto-complete feature, barcode scanner of medicines and an intelligent AI-based chatbot were incorporated innovatively in the second version of the prototype developed by the next batch of Capstone students in a Scrum-based project management paradigm. Figure 4 provides the screenshots of the second prototype which predominantly satisfied the CAM consumer needs.

Essential to the effectiveness of the App, was ensuring the design, production and functional requirements of the IMgateway Consumer App were user led, was essential to the effectiveness of the App (Eyles et al. 2016; Venkatraman 2017; Anderson et al. 2016). Subsequent to the inclusion of community input that was translated into project designs and prototypes, the iterative development of the

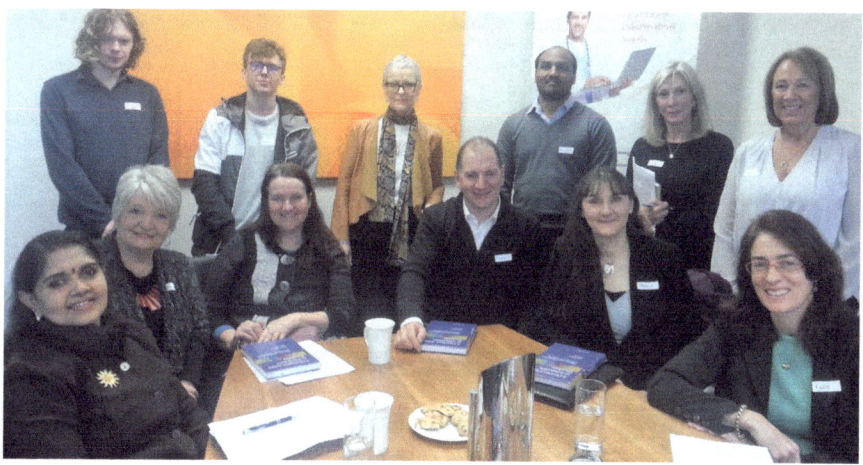

Fig. 2 Consumer-led, co-designed research project meeting. L-R Dr. Sitalakshmi Venkatraman (Melbourne Polytechnic), Caiden Brandon (Student, Melbourne Polytechnic), Tricia Greenway (Community Engagement Adviser), Jakub Suplicki (Student, Melbourne Polytechnic), Jane Scoble (BCNA), Late Sally Percival Wood, Peter De Lorenzo (UnityHealth), Amar Erigela (UnityHealth), Dr Vesna Grubacevic (PhD Cl Hyp), Keryn Coghill (Pharmacist), Leslie Gilham (BCNA) and Professor Kylie O'Brien (Adjunct Professor Torrens University, Adjunct Fellow NICM Health Research Centre, Western Sydney University))

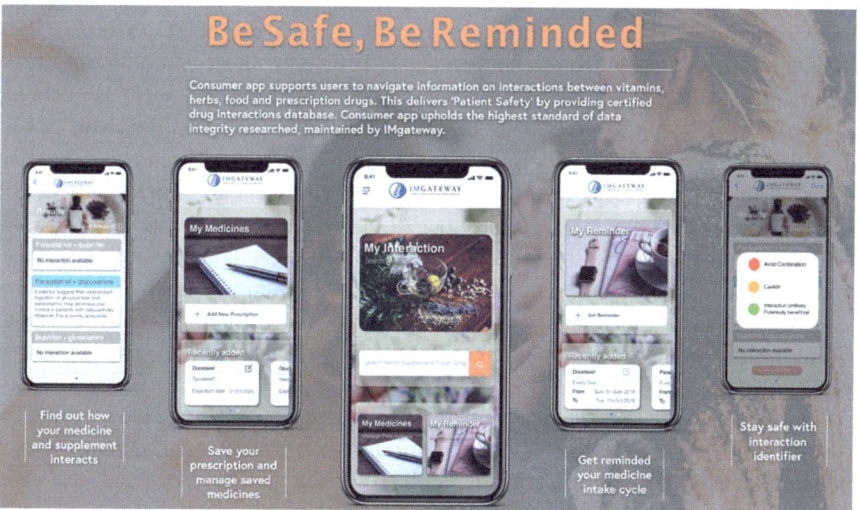

Fig. 3 First prototype of IMgateway Consumer App

prototype underwent testing by consumer groups, and the feedback led to product adaptation and retesting. Overall, the App aims to enhance consumer confidence to share CAM information with their health professionals through IMgateway and its collaborative mainstream drug information system partners. The information can

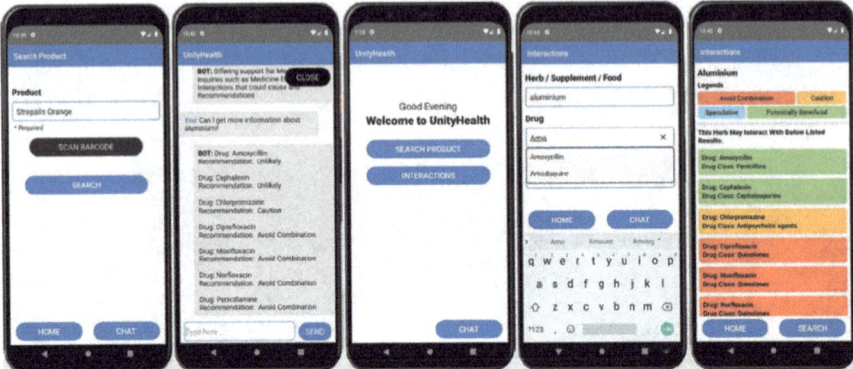

Fig. 4 Second prototype of IMgateway Consumer App

also now be made readily available on mobile platforms for patients and their care-givers. The end users of this project include all clinical professionals and their patients, and members of the public who avail themselves of off-the-shelf drugs, and traditional Chinese and complementary medicines. This body of users comprises a large fraction of the population of Victoria in Australia.

Currently, there is no readily available advice on ADRs between drugs and traditional Chinese or complementary medicines. Such a service will provide an educative link between patients, customers and clinicians that will increase the understanding of patients and thereby strengthen engagement of customers with their clinicians. Strengthened engagement will deliver effective communication, accuracy of treatments and management of chronic diseases, such as diabetes (Tricco et al. 2012; Castelnuovo et al. 2015; Schmitt et al. 2013; Dawson 2017). Together, these benefits will deliver reduced morbidity and reduced health service costs. The IMgateway Consumer App will translate the clinical advice of UnityHealth's IMgateway to 'consumer friendly' advice for the patient. The IMgateway Consumer App is now in the Prototype Development and Evaluation phase. It is envisaged that eventually our proposed system will address all interactions between prescribed and over-the-counter drugs, and food, and traditional and Chinese and complementary medicines, for which sufficient peer reviewed evidence is available.

In the past couple of years, the COVID-19 pandemic has changed the way healthcare is routinely delivered worldwide. In particular, the Retail Pharmacy sector which is one of the key IM stakeholders in Australia and New Zealand, has been greatly impacted. Pharmacists have increasingly taken a lead role in meeting individual patient needs across practice settings (Worley 2006; Harnett et al. 2018; Popatti et al. 2018; Harnett et al. 2018). Community pharmacists have also continued to serve patients throughout the pandemic by increasing the accessibility of medications via curbside and home delivery services. Furthermore, their knowledge in IM would help support additional roles to serve patients including—the increased use of telehealth to provide continuous care in office-based practices in clinics, in community pharmacies, as well as in COVID-19 testing and vaccination efforts. These changes have impacted the pharmacy workforce with low rates of staff retention in Pharmacy (Rx) retail stores, with a growing number of pharmacists leaving the profession due to 'burn out'. While Government and Universities would seek to graduate more students to support the future needs of the community; UnityHealth has proactively launched another project to address the needs of the pharmacy workforce.

The Rx store owners and Rx banner group head office management seek the right mix of staff skills to support their customers. Most experts agree that a patient-centred approach to healthcare is the most effective approach and ongoing training in Rx customer service and quality use of medicines is vitally important within our multicultural society. Because of this, store owners seek improved, up to date insights into how their workforce is equipped to serve the community (Ung et al. 2018). They will identify the gaps in staff skills and train and recruit staff to ensure the business runs as an efficient, local health destination for improved community health, thereby reducing healthcare costs incurred by individuals and the government (Lee et al. 2018; Australian Institute of Health and Welfare 2018b; Twigg 2019). In this project, we aim to study the pharmacy workforce needs in the next 3 years. We make use of UnityHealth's e-learning platform iTherapeutics (www. iTherapeutics.com.au) that provides online training, including CAM for pharmacists and pharmacy assistants in Australia as shown in Fig. 5. Using such an e-learning platform, the project's goal is to provide the Rx Store Owner the knowledge and business intelligence (BI) to plan, implement and monitor staff training and skills/qualifications, against the health needs of the local community. All information requirements of Rx education will be sourced from the iTherapeutics' database. With the community population statistics sourced from the Australian Government's ABS website, iTherapeutics and other tools will be used to survey Rx staff and study their responses to key questions. The survey data collected will be studied for trends and gaps analysis. The data insights and Business Intelligence reports will be accessible by Rx store owners via secure login to the iTherapeutics website. The first deliverable will be to complete a detailed requirements analysis in

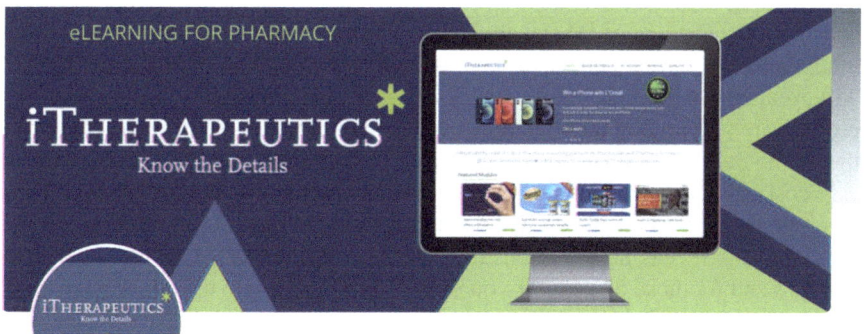

Fig. 5 iTherapeutics—e-learning platform for pharmacy

order to meet the needs of Rx store owners. We believe that our collaborative research in IM supports the national strategic pathway to achieve the most appropriate care for each person (Langevin 2021).

4   Conclusions and Future Work

This chapter provided a summary of our journey and the positive impact in IM that has been delivered through research and IT innovations. With the upsurge in the use of complementary medicine and the recent healthcare challenges posed by the COVID-19 pandemic, key IT projects and innovative application developments enhanced the applicability of UnityHealth's IMgateway and iTherapeutics. The projects' requirements for clinical expertise, system engineering, IT research and development and marketing were well satisfied with a balance of skills afforded by collaboration among UnityHealth partners.

Our contributions are mainly threefold. Firstly, our pursuit of better health has been made possible through consumer-led IM initiatives leading to innovative IT projects. The projects have leveraged the latest advances in IT such as data analytics, cloud computing, GPS enablement, AI and mobile computing. Secondly, the foundation has been built using science-based resources, developed over the last two decades, that are regularly updated by academia and professional bodies in IM. The Imgateway database is broadly used and accessible by healthcare professionals via Drug Info Systems, MIMS (https://www.mims.com.au/) and AusDI (https://www.ausdi.com/). Thirdly, UnityHealth projects have been co-designed to meet the needs of all stakeholders. There has been no pharmaceutical advertising or funding to date, and our project implementations are based on consumer group recommendations and the support of consumer forum groups, using an Agile project management method.

Currently, UnityHealth is on the advisory board of several IM committees. Its health information services and the online educative process via its e-Learning platforms and user-friendly Apps, will lead to better health literacy, training and engagement among the public, clinical professionals and the pharmacy workforce. An enhanced engagement of IM stakeholders will deliver more accurate diagnoses and more appropriate treatments and the community's enhanced knowledge of ADRs will eventually reduce morbidity and health care costs. In summary, these ongoing projects are poised to make a significant contribution to the emerging health policy theme of 'Self-Care'. In particular the need to address adverse events and health care costs by minimising avoidable medicine interactions and subsequent hospital admissions, visits to the doctor and ADR fatalities.

Victoria's citizens have demonstrated a ready acceptance of mobile ICT technologies and for those 65 years or younger, mobile devices are the preferred method of communication. For the more senior citizens, there is still extensive demand for conventional ICT technologies. Accordingly, the needs of the entire customer base will be better met by providing a mix of technological and digital channels. Future work will firstly consider the delivery of an Open General Site that will provide the public with access to clinical advice on herb/ supplement/food-drug interactions through keyword searches. Documents that have been conditioned for easy reading in non-technical language will be presented in standard text format suitable for access on PCs, mobile phones, tablets and eReaders. Consumer experiences, reports on ADRs and reports related to chronic disease management and wellness will be made available. Consumers will be able to access their specific circumstance-based drug interaction information and links to relevant specialists. Secondly, an Open Reference Site will permit access to a restricted range of peer-reviewed references that are closely targeted to the patient's concerns, including ADRs. Consumers will be led by keyword search to appropriately validated references. Thirdly, a Specialist Site will provide secure communication between medical practitioners, pharmacists and other clients that will ensure more personalised and effective treatments. By having patients and end users involved during the design and production phases of prototype development, the effectiveness of solutions will be ensured.

References

Anderson K, et al. Mobile health apps to facilitate self-care. PLoS One. 2016;11(5):e0156164.

Australian Bureau of Statistics. National health survey: persons. 2020.

Australian Commission on Safety and Quality in Health Care. Quality use of medicines and medicines safety discussion paper. 2020. https://www.safetyandquality.gov.au/publications-and-resources/resource-library/quality-use-medicines-and-medicines-safety-discussion-paper.

Australian Institute of Health and Welfare. Hospital performance: costs of acute admitted patients in public hospitals from 2012-13 to 2014-15. Canberra: AIHW; 2018a.

Australian Institute of Health and Welfare. Australia's health 2018: in brief. Cat. no. AUS 222. Canberra: AIHW; 2018b.

Australian Institute of Health and Welfare. Health expenditure Australia 2018–2019. 2020. https://www.aihw.gov.au/reports/health-welfare-expenditure/health-expenditure-australia-2018-19/contents/summary.

BMA British Medical Association. Report on complementary medicine: new approaches to good practice. Oxford: Oxford University Press; 1993.

Castelnuovo G, et al. New technologies for the management of rehabilitation of chronic diseases and conditions. Biomed Res Int. 2015;2015:180436.

CMA Complementary Medicines Australia. Pre-budget submission 2020-21. 2022. Accessed https://www.cmaustralia.org.au/resources/Documents/CMA%20Pre-Budget%20Submission%202021-22%20Submitted%20(for%20website).pdf.

Commonwealth of Australia. Australian Bureau of Statistics, National Health Survey: First Results, 2017-18. 2019.

Dawson W. Differential relationships between diabetes knowledge scales and diabetes outcomes. Diabetes Educ. 2017;43(4):360–6.

De Lorenzo P. Bridging the gap with the integration of conventional and complementary medicine. Middle East J Family Med. 2007;5:2.

Easton K, Morgan T, Williamson M. Medication safety in the community: a review of the literature. Sydney: National Prescribing Service; 2009.

Edwards IR, Aronson JK. Adverse drug reactions: definitions, diagnosis, and management. Lancet. 2000;356(9237):1255–9.

Eyles H, et al. Co-design of mHealth delivered interventions: a systematic review to assess key methods and processes. Curr Nutr Rep. 2016;5(3):160–7.

Gallego G, Gugnani S, Armour M, Smith CA, Chang E. Attitudes and factors involved in decision-making around complementary and alternative medicines (CAMs) by older Australians: a qualitative study. Eur J Integr Med. 2019;29:100930.

Greenstock L, et al. Telecommunications and health information for culturally and linguistically diverse communities: a community survey. Telecommun J Austr. 2013;63(1):1–18.

Harnett J, Le TQ, Smith L, Krass I. Perceptions, opinions and knowledge of pharmacists towards the use of complementary medicines by people living with cancer. Int J Clin Pharm. 2018;40(5):1272–80.

Huang Z, et al. Medication management support in diabetes: a systematic assessment of diabetes self-management apps. BMC Med. 2019;17:127.

Langevin HM. NCCIH strategic plan FY 2021–2025: mapping a pathway to research on whole person health. National Center for Complementary and Integrative Health website. 2021. https://www.nccih.nih.gov/about/nccih-strategic-plan-2021-2025.

Lee CMY, Goode B, Nørtoft E, Shaw JE, Magliano DJ, Colagiuri S. The cost of diabetes and obesity in Australia. J Med Econ. 2018;21(10):1001–5.

Ng JY. The regulation of complementary and alternative medicine professions in Ontario, Canada. Integr Med Res. 2020;9(1):12–6.

Ng JY, Mooghali M, Munford V. eHealth technologies assisting in identifying potential adverse interactions with complementary and alternative medicine (CAM) or standalone CAM adverse events or side effects: a scoping review. BMC Complementary Med Ther. 2020;20(1):1–26.

O'Brien K, Moore A, Percival-Smith S, Venkatraman S, Grubacevic V, Scoble J, Gilham L, Greenway T, Coghill K, Wale J. An investigation into the usability of a drug-complementary medicines interactions database in a consumer group of women with breast cancer. Eur J Integr Med. 2020;33:1–9.

Popatti A, et al. Ethical responsibilities of pharmacists when selling CMs: a systematic review. Int J Pharm Pract. 2018;26(2):93–103.

PSA Pharmaceutical Society of Australia. Medicine safety: take care. Canberra: PSA; 2019.

Schmid O, Bereznicki B, Peterson GM, Stankovich J, Bereznicki L. Persistence of adverse drug reaction-related hospitalization risk following discharge. Int J Environ Res Public Health. 2022;19:5585.

Schmitt A, et al. The Diabetes Self-Management Questionnaire (DSMQ): development and evaluation of an instrument to assess diabetes self-care activities associated with glycaemic control. Health Qual Life Outcomes. 2013;11:1138.

Steel A, McIntyre E, Harnett J, et al. Complementary medicine use in the Australian population: results of a nationally-representative cross-sectional survey. Sci Rep. 2018;8:17325.

Strand LM, et al. Drug-related problems: their structure and function. Drug Intell Clin Pharm. 1990;24(11):1093–7.

Tricco AC, et al. Effectiveness of quality improvement strategies on the management of diabetes: a systematic review and meta-analysis. Lancet. 2012;379(9833):2252–61.

Twigg W. The pharmacy care plan service: evaluation and estimate of cost-effectiveness. Res Soc Adm Pharm. 2019;15(1):84–92.

Ung COL, Harnett J, Hu H. Development of a strategic model for integrating complementary medicines into professional pharmacy practice. Res Soc Adm Pharm. 2018;14(7):663–72.

Venkatraman S. User-centric ontology for smart holistic health information systems. IJSMR. 2017;3:23–37.

Venkatraman S, Stranieri A. Unification of electronic health records and CAM. In: Proceedings of 3rd International Conference on Holistic Medicine. Colombo: ICHM; 2012.

von Conrady DM, Bonney A. Patterns of complementary and alternative medicine use and health literacy in general practice patients in urban and regional, Australia. Aust Fam Physician. 2017;46(5):316–20.

World Health Organization. Regional Office for the Western Pacific. Regional framework for harnessing traditional and complementary medicine for achieving health and well-being in the Western Pacific. WHO Regional Office for the Western Pacific. 2022. https://apps.who.int/iris/handle/10665/355150.

Worley MM. Testing a pharmacist-patient relationship quality model among older persons with diabetes. Res Soc Adm Pharm. 2006;2(1):1–21.

Peter De Lorenzo is the founding Director of UnityHealth Pty Ltd His unique and broad experience in the healthcare industry spans over 40 years in both business and information technology projects. After 20 years in the Corporate Business and IT industry, (beginning with The Australian Bank), he was onboarded to Partner at Deloitte Consulting Australia in the late 90s. Peter successfully established UnityHealth and pioneered the strategy, design and implementation of the first Australian based, Integrative Medicine portal IMgateway.net in 2001. Over the years, UnityHealth has successfully established active and strategic working partnerships with the University of Sydney, the National Institute of Complementary Medicine at the Western Sydney University, MIMS Drug Information Systems, Melbourne Polytechnic and a large range of multi-national clients.

UnityHealth is an independent digital health information, education and technology services Company that aims to empower practitioners and consumers to combine high quality, evidence-based interventions to achieve the best possible health outcomes. We accomplish this through the provision of our leading online education resources, IMgateway and iTherapeutics, as well as our active working partnerships with leading organisations.

Sitalakshmi Venkatraman is a Senior Lecturer in the Department of Information Technology at Melbourne Polytechnic. Sita has more than 30 years of rich international work experience in academics and industry. She has taught a variety of IT courses at the postgraduate and undergraduate levels for tertiary institutions in India, Singapore, New Zealand, and Australia. Currently at Melbourne Polytechnic she is the Discipline Leader of Business Analytics and coordinates Industry Capstone Projects. Sita's recent research predominantly focuses on proposing and evaluating models and frameworks for industry problems from various domains, the data mining, e-health and e-security specialised topics related to personalised healthcare. She has considered social and technological risks and privacy/security issues in the design and evaluation of user-centric information system in her research problems. Her contribution to UnityHealth projects include the design, implementation, and evaluation towards enhancing their digital platforms (eHealth sites and mHealth apps).

My Personal, Professional, and Academic Journey and Lived Experience with Domestic Violence

Leo Brunelle

Abstract Regardless of its definition or perception, intimate partner, domestic, or family violence is a crime and remains a societal scourge around the world. Some people grow up in loving, stable homes while others are raised in an environment filled with violence, rage, fear, dysfunction, and toxicity. In the household I was raised in, discipline always came in the form of verbal and physical violence which was considered "the norm." My personal development from infancy and into early adulthood was chaotic and destructive and I had no positive male role model in my life. I became needy, insecure, nihilistic, and angry with everyone and everything around me; I constantly failed in my own intimate and personal relationships.

Academically, I was a below average student; professionally, I was undereducated with no advancement potential and I faced a life of perpetual failure. Now, upon reflection, I am convinced that my lived experience with domestic violence very nearly doomed me a cycle of failure. When I became a police officer, I used my personal experience with domestic violence to empathize with the victim; to be her champion. My goal was to become that officer who understood domestic violence, to bring her abuser to justice, and free her from being constantly abused. Later in my policing career, I wanted to transfer that personal and professional knowledge into a doctoral study and become a respected scholar/practitioner.

Keywords Domestic violence · Lived experience · Personal · Professional · Academic · Toxic · Chaotic · Dysfunctional

L. Brunelle (✉)
Institute for Innovation Science and Sustainability, Federation University, Mt. Helen, VIC, Australia
e-mail: l.brunelle@federation.edu.au

© The Author(s), under exclusive license to Springer Nature Singapore Pte Ltd. 2024
A. Stranieri et al. (eds.), *Research Partners with Lived Experience*,
https://doi.org/10.1007/978-981-97-0033-2_9

1   Introduction

I have never understood why violence in the home or an intimate relationship was and is still considered a personal, private family affair. It seems that few people are willing to get involved to stop or prevent an act of violence and to protect the victim. This singular question remains: "How does anyone justify using violence, abuse, and intimidation against another person or family member they claim to love?" Anyone, male or female, who resorts to the use of violence, in any form, solely intended to dominate or intimidate is a coward. Abusive and violent people possess inherent insecurities such as: anger, fear, and rage; they demonstrate little empathy toward other human beings and animals.

Personally, my perspective is that violence is the tool of an undeveloped mind, an individual with low EQ [1]; incapable of expressing any empathy. I despise violent people; they serve no purpose in civilized society and I believe that domestic violence underpins the barbarity we see publicly. If you wonder why a kid bullies another kid, shows cruelty to an animal, take a look at his or her home life. Boys are still taught that toughness and respect are gained through the use of violence and yes, girls are taught the same lesson. If one is disrespected, mocked, or there is a disagreement, the use of violence is justified to regain "honor" or make a point. My father used violence to enforce "discipline," suppress disagreement or expression; his word, his will, and his "knowledge" were never to be questioned. In his mind, he was the supreme authority in the house and for anyone to express displeasure or disagreement paid a heavy price. I did not have the ability to have a discourse with anyone out of fear of being a victim of physical violence or retaliation. My story is my lived experience with domestic violence on a personal, professional, and academic level; I do not seek pity, only understanding. My story intends for the reader to view this phenomenon from a different lens, that is, largely misunderstood, especially among many police officers. My intent was to take my personal and professional lived experience with domestic violence and transfer that knowledge gained into a doctoral thesis.

2   My Personal Lived Experience with Domestic Violence

I was born in September 1958, the eldest of five boys, and my father was career military; my mom, she stayed at home. The stereotypical American family during the 1950s, 1960s, and 1970s consisted of a mother and a father and x number of children. This was the era in I grew up in, moving from one base to another every three years and never putting down roots. Despite my description of what was

---

[1] EQ is defined as emotional quotient, a (notional) measure of a person's adequacy in such areas as self- awareness, empathy, and dealing sensitively with other people (Collins English Dictionary 2014).

considered "typical," we were not what was depicted in the American television show "Leave it to Beaver." This iconic series was set in the 1950s, in an idealistic two parent home with two children, a father, the breadwinner, and a mother, the homemaker. Family problems and discipline involved conversations that were always gentle and both parents would give sage advice ending in an unrealistically happy resolution. The home and familial environment that my mom, my brothers, and I lived in was toxic, violent, chaotic, and dysfunctional; it was hell.

During the 1960s and 1970s, in the military and civilian settings I grew up in, I never saw police respond to domestic violence. The mentality during that time was that no one intervened; if the police did respond, they could or would do little to nothing. Throughout 1967, my father would come home from the NCO [2] club completely intoxicated and would immediately proceed to vent his rage at everyone. If me or one of my brothers were in arm's reach, he would grab and shake us violently, while yelling in our faces. He would mercilessly scream at my mom and point out every single fault, real or imagined, while we all sat helplessly and cried. In 1969, I once saw him grab my mom, hold her hands together and slap her during an argument, I could do nothing. In my 11-year-old mind, I wished I had a gun, because I would have shot him dead and ended the violence. No one called the base police, no one came to my mom's aid; only a neighbor kid came to watch and he laughed. He did not laugh for long as two of my brothers and I proceeded to beat him, only his screams stopped my father. He came running outside, demanding what had happened, I told him this punk kid was laughing at him slapping mom and he froze.

He then got into our Volkswagen van and drove off back to the NCO club where he had gotten drunk earlier that morning. We were living in Puerto Rico then; my mom had no one to call and she would never call her family for help. My mom had no job skills, only a high school education, no driver's license, and the family lived paycheck to paycheck. There was no way she could leave with five young boys in tow and she had nowhere to go; she was trapped. The incident was never reported because of the extreme risk of substantial disciplinary action or court-martial to my father by his commanding officer. My father had been disciplined four times previously for driving while intoxicated and each time resulted in him having been reduced in rank. I suspect that a fifth time would have resulted in him being forced into retirement with 24 years [3] already served on active duty. They "reconciled" and oddly enough, he never hit her again; but the ongoing alcohol and verbal abuse coupled with his drunken outbursts continued. My father retired from the military in 1973 and until his death in 1996, he drifted in and out of minimum wage jobs. I struggled throughout high school and barely graduated; I had enlisted 6 months prior and I was passed just to get me out. I enlisted in the military to escape the family because I felt that I was a financial burden and another mouth to feed. My father

---

[2] NCO is an abbreviation for "non-commissioned officer" in the American military of rankings E4 to E9.

[3] In the US military, a member must serve for 20 years before becoming eligible for retirement.

informed me that there was no money for college and I would have to join the military or go to work.

I opted to enlist because the military had an educational program for honorably discharged or retired veterans; it was the only option available. I was in a situation where I had no job skills, no job, and no money to go to college; I felt trapped. My mom begged me not to enlist, she said I was too young, and I was too immature for life in the military. I disregarded her advice; she reluctantly signed the enlistment forms and my father gladly signed, which became a mistake I would later regret. Because I scored low in the aptitude tests for jobs in the Air Force, I was placed into a job I absolutely hated. I cross-trained four years later into Security Police because I had always wanted to be a police officer and I extended my enlistment. At the time, it seemed like a good idea, fulfilling my new commitment and then transitioning into civilian life as a civilian cop. Unfortunately, my dysfunctional and immature behavior made it obvious that I was unsuited for military life and I was discharged in 1981. My mom's prophecy eventuated and I found myself back to square one: living at home and back into the same environment I fled. But it was different this time, my middle brother had died 2 years prior, my father was working overseas, and I was lost.

For the next 3 years, I drifted in and out of jobs, exhausted my military educational benefits and still had no career path. I finally found a steady job, got married, saved enough money to buy a house; finding the stability in my life I craved. In 1989, I completed my associate's degree and wanted to complete my bachelor's but raising a family on a single income prevented that. In 1991, I was informed that I had 2 years to complete college or trade school for a different position within the organization. I decided that I was stable and mature enough to go back into law enforcement and went to my youngest brother for help. He was a sergeant with a local police department and had all of the connections to get me sponsored into the police academy. My application was accepted and in January 1993, I worked full-time during the day and attended the police academy 8 hours a night. I graduated in April 1993 and for the next 6 months, I submitted applications to different law enforcement organizations hoping to get hired. In October 1993, I finally was offered a position with a small Central Florida police department where I would spend my entire 15-year police career. I was 12 years older, emotionally settled, far more responsible; and I was much better educated; I was ready and determined to succeed. Domestic violence response and intervention was an interest early in my career where I wanted to excel, but I had much to learn. Rookie police officers fresh out of the academy often have misguided ideas of saving the world and throwing the bad guys in jail.

I held a very naïve, idealistic, and completely unrealistic mindset that the good citizens would embrace my noble, altruistic intent with open arms. When it came to domestic violence response and intervention, that illusion was immediately shattered, and reality became a rude wake-up call for me. I soon discovered that not all female victims of domestic violence are grateful or cooperative, and not all of the offenders are compliant. Regardless of what was taught in the academy and field training, putting into practical application what one learns is most often diametrically opposed. Despite my detailed reports, collection of physical evidence, sworn statements from witnesses and the victim, the end result fell short of my expectations. Victims often recanted their stories and defended the abuser; the State Attorney's Office would drop the case or would offer a plea deal. Personally, I took that as an affront to my efforts to help the victim and hold the abuser accountable, why was this happening? Professionally, I was about to embark on a long and difficult journey toward better understanding the dynamics and intricate complexities of domestic violence.

3 My Professional Lived Experience with Domestic Violence

The academic and theoretical elements of what a police academy cadet learns often differs greatly into what happens in a real-life application. Unfortunately, I was horribly naïve and idealistic; possessing a "save the world" mentality and I very quickly learned that this was a folly. I once held unrealistic virtuous and selfless notions toward becoming that one police officer who would be the "hero" to an abused woman. I took on face value what I was taught by my academy instructors and the statutory guidelines and criminal laws of the state. I was not prepared to address or understand the "gray areas," or nuances when dealing with the variety of issues I would face. When it came to domestic violence intervention, I discovered that abusers and victims often did not react what was taught in the textbooks. In my mind, she would be eternally grateful, would leave her abusive spouse, and would live happily ever after; I was sadly mistaken. Police academy instructors teach a lot of theory and often regale police cadets with "war stories" into how they caught the bad guys (Prokos and Padavic 2002). Academically, theory is fine, it provides an underpinning into the foundation of learning, but reality is the true teacher and it is brutal. Watching old videos of how to intervene in domestic violence calls and role-play pales in comparison to a real-life dynamic and unpredictable event. I learned quickly that theory and reality are not aligned when dealing with a violent, intoxicated suspect and a distraught and histrionic victim.

I also discovered that some abused women would suddenly turn on you and rarely reciprocated their gratitude for your efforts, compassion, and understanding. I found that my efforts were often in vain and I would be back at the same house again with the same actors. I have had veteran officers and sergeants show me their scars from knife attacks from battered women "defending" their abusers from being arrested. What I failed to understand for a long time was just how complicated intervening and addressing domestic violence cases are for police officers. In academy and field training, rookie officers are taught technical and legal skills, departmental policies and procedures in domestic violence response, nothing more.

They are trained to act in this sequence:

1. A two unit response, arriving quickly and silently.
2. Park two houses away, making a quiet approach on foot.

3. Visually observing and listening carefully.
4. Looking in windows while listening for signs of fighting, yelling, or crying.
5. Announce your presence, providing the residents an opportunity to answer.
6. If the parties refuse to open the door or fail to respond, make entry into the house. [4]
7. Secure and separate the parties, conduct a protective sweep of the house for others.
8. Secure the scene and notifying emergency medical services.
9. Render first aid and begin the investigation.

This was the response protocol guided by Florida State constitutional and criminal statutory guidelines, traffic laws, and police agency departmental policies and procedures (Domestic Relations 2021; Lake Mary Police Department 2018). Besides responding and intervening, collecting evidence, determining the primary aggressor, and arresting the suspect when probable cause was established, nothing more was done. The position of my agency with domestic violence response was what I previously described and went back into service as soon as possible. There are three avenues police departments take when probable cause exists in a domestic violence to effect an arrest: mandatory, preferred, and discretionary (Hirschel 2009; Lake Mary Police Department 2018).

All law enforcement organizations in Florida are mandated with the preferred arrest policy: when probable cause exists, the preferred response is to arrest. This approach was predicated by a watershed high court decision of Thurman v City of Torrington (Thurman v. City of Torrington 1984) forever changed police response to domestic violence. [5] Domestic violence training for police to "accurately" identify a primary aggressor was a nebulous, subjective, and problematic approach that often failed female victims. Too many women were arrested because of inaccurate and misleading information complicated by indifferent police officers who were pressured to clear the call. I unreservedly admit that my limited knowledge of domestic violence response was quite poor and based upon my police academy and field training. Early in my career, I made the mistake of arresting several female victims after taking on face value the allegation of their abusers. I attribute my lack of critical thinking skills and inadequate training leading to these egregious acts where I had unknowingly revictimized the victim. Other external elements beyond my control contributed to my convoluted and seemingly lack of understanding into domestic violence response, further complicating my comprehension.

I had adopted the mentality of "she deserves what she gets if she goes back," despite what I had been taught in training. I became cynical, myopic, and distrustful

---

[4] Under Florida law, entry into a home may be made under exigent circumstances to prevent further injury or the suspect from obtaining a weapon. Officers may make a protective sweep of the residence to locate injured or deceased persons or children hiding. Officers must make a clear and loud announcement when entering.

[5] In Torrington, Connecticut, 1984, the Torrington Police Department was successfully sued by Tracy Thurman for their failure in protecting her from her abusive husband. This was the impetus in changing you police organizations responded to domestic violence calls.

of victims and responding to domestic violence calls became an effort in futility, why should I bother?

When I attended an advanced domestic violence intervention course, I voiced that misguided opinion and during a break my instructor pulled me aside. She was highly regarded and an experienced domestic violence victim's advocate and proceeded to privately give me a well- deserved and proper dressing down. She informed me of the reasons why many victims recant and why they act the way they do with police in these cases. She told me that if I could or would not comprehend what she was teaching, I would continue to do more considerable harm. I did notice that I was the only male police officer she took aside despite that there were other men in the class. I was not the only one who vocalized this attitude, but I was the only one this instructor pulled up and spoke to. Upon reflection, this became a teachable moment for me where I needed to readjust my lens into how I viewed domestic violence intervention.

I took to heart what she told me, and I listened to her more attentively, taking a different perspective in domestic violence response. If I were to become that police officer I aspired to be and to evolve professionally, I had to make some significant changes. After that, I became more determined toward taking a more progressive approach in how I responded to, investigated, and processed domestic violence cases. I began to take an academic approach by reading publications into the dynamics and complexities of domestic violence from experts in the field. For the next several years, I compared and contrasted the theoretical and academic applications to what I experienced real-time while in the field. I began to gain a better and deeper understanding into domestic violence and developed my critical thinking skills toward a more evolved viewpoint. It became my objective to design and create a more progressive protocol and approach to improve how police respond to domestic violence cases. At that time, I was very fortunate that I had a transformative command staff who were quite supportive with my efforts and project. Unfortunately, I did not receive the desired support from many of my peers, line supervisors or some senior staff and it became frustrating.

I was subjected to ridicule and criticism, being regarded as taking a foolish pursuit that was considered as "social work," not "real" policing. The essence of policing is underpinned by hegemonic and hyper masculine behaviors and mindsets and transcends the entirety of a law enforcement organization (Cooper 2009; Prokos and Padavic 2002). These behaviors and attitudes became the impetus for me to continue what I was doing because I was determined to prove them wrong. I took the opportunity to become a state certified police trainer where I could conduct in-house training for police and criminal justice professionals. I was taught how to construct, design, and develop a living training curriculum with learning objectives and learning outcomes underpinned by published scholarship. I conducted training within my own and my brother's departments, and to judges, domestic violence advocates, child and elder protection practioners, women's groups, and conferences. My professional education did not stop there, I proceeded to complete my academic pursuit of bachelor's and master's degrees in 2002 and 2004. I began the process of combining my professional and academic experiences to supplement my overall knowledge into the training programs I was creating. To me, it became very important to blend the academic scholarship with the pragmatic approach in how police respond to domestic violence cases. I was not a true academic but was becoming a practitioner scholar providing a clearer understanding and practical application into domestic violence response (Workman 2007).

Being an insider researcher and creating an understandable learning platform to line staff, while not insulting their intelligence was reaping more positive results (Workman 2007). While I still faced resistance from older officers who still retained 'old school' attitudes, the approach was viewed as transformative to newer officers. Between 1997 and 2002, I was assigned to the undercover narcotics and vice task force and my work on domestic violence was suspended. During that time, I worked a drug case that involved a young woman who was a victim of domestic violence that ended badly. This became an event that haunts me to this very day and it is one I will never forget; I still blame myself. I was tasked with investigating prescription fraud cases and received a call from a local pharmacist of a case of a forged prescription. After talking with the pharmacist and the physician it was confirmed that this particular prescription was a fake, so I sat and waited. After a 30 minute wait, my suspect arrived; a twenty something woman, very attractive and petite; initially, her appearance was unremarkable which surprised me. In previous encounters with suspects, they presented certain behaviors: looking around for a uniformed officer and acting very skittish; she exhibited no trepidation.

When the transaction was completed, I approached this young woman, presented my credentials, informed her of the situation, and placed her under arrest. After taking her to the Sheriff's Office substation, I made contact with her husband and soon discovered that she was being abused. He became very angry and threatening with me when I informed him of the circumstances and requested him to come get their car. I immediately informed him that he would not continue speaking to me this way and he had 30 minutes to come collect his car. He was more concerned about the car than his wife and told me to "leave her in fucking jail"; he did not care. He showed up 15 minutes later, was given the keys to the car, and informed my supervisor that I had "a shit attitude." My supervisor laughed at him and said that he had no problem with the way I handled the situation, telling him to leave. It became apparent to me that this young woman was self-medicating to manage her anxiety and depression because of her husband's ongoing abuse. I told her that I could and would help her by referring her to a local safehouse that would provide counseling for her. I said that I would recommend to the State Attorney to get her into rehabilitation and in touch with the domestic violence division. Before I had her transported to jail, I gave her my business card to call me any time if she needed help. This proved to be futile because a year later, I received a call from another pharmacy that she had passed another forged prescription. When I pulled into the shopping mall parking lot, I saw her walking to her car with an unexpected surprise: she was pregnant.

I was very upset that when I saw her it was very obvious that she was very close to her delivery due date. I was again faced with a dilemma: arrest a heavily pregnant woman, she goes into labor and delivers the baby while in custody. I was not concerned about the optics of or any political fallout from a media frenzy, I was simply not going to arrest her. One thing I learned in the academy and in the field, police officers are given latitude to exercise discretion in certain exigent circumstances. This became an example of being creative while still being legally compliant with state statutory and agency policies, so I called my supervisor. I presented my proposal and he was neither impressed nor happy with my recommendation: confiscate the bottle of pills and complete a capias. [6] I explained that she was close to giving birth and not wanting the Sheriff's Office to incur the cost of an in-custody birth. He reluctantly acquiesced and allowed me to place the pills into evidentiary control and complete the capias; I did and sent her home. I told her that I hoped that she had not taken any pills during her pregnancy for the health of her unborn baby. It would be the last time I ever saw her in person; she gave birth to a healthy baby girl 2 weeks later.

Six weeks following the baby's birth, she was arrested; I had never seen that kind of turnaround for any minor felony drug charge. Six months later, I returned to the uniformed division as a new sergeant and received a phone call from a buddy of mine. He asked me if I remembered this young woman and I told him that I did and immediately asked him what was wrong. He told me she had been found by her husband earlier that day hanging in the garage, appearing that she had committed suicide. I was devastated; thinking to myself I should have taken the bottle, put her into my vehicle, and drove her to the safehouse. I had connections and should have not been so focused on making an arrest; I was so angry with my incredibly stupid decision. Her husband was initially under suspicion by investigators for possibly murdering her and making it look like suicide, but an investigation exonerated him. Several months later, while having breakfast, I noticed someone walking up to me and it was a lieutenant I had worked for previously. He asked if he could sit with me and told me that he wanted to talk to me, and I asked him why. He told me that he knew what happened to this young woman and was concerned about me having taken her death so hard. I told him that I felt completely responsible for the stupid decision I made and felt that I could have done things differently.

He looked at me and said that in no way was I responsible, punctuating that I tried harder than anyone else would have. He told me that I had correctly assessed the problem and had offered her every opportunity to reach out and accept my help. I told him that I had difficulty accepting that point of view and that I should have done a lot more for her. He told me that the decision to take me up on those offers was hers and hers alone and that I was not responsible. He left me with this comment: "Sometimes, despite your best efforts, you cannot and will never save everyone"; I still felt no better. To this day, I have not reconciled this and I have never forgiven myself and it is a spectre that will eternally haunt me.

---

[6] A capias is request submitted to the State Attorney's Office for misdemeanor drug or non-violent crimes. This was a situation where this was a third-degree felony, the lowest category of felonies. Filing this request was a reasonable avenue in this situation and is not commonly done.

4   My Academic Lived Experience with Domestic Violence

In 2006, I decided to undertake a doctoral project on police response to incidents of domestic violence, combining my personal and professional experiences. I wanted to research and examine why law enforcement organizations and their officers were still not responding to domestic violence appropriately or efficiently. I had developed several theories into why this was and wanted to explore these hypotheses more closely toward constructing a more holistic approach. I developed three theories based upon my professional training, education, and field experience responding to domestic violence calls: (a) training and education, (b) organizational structure and issues of masculinity, and (c) leadership, supervision, organizational policies and procedures. Reflecting upon my own professional experiences responding to and intervening in incidents of domestic violence, I compared them to those of other officers. I discovered that formal intervention by police into domestic violence was one of a multitude of responses involving a variety of different stakeholders.

Responding to domestic violence cases is not binary or black and white; domestic violence is extremely complicated and beyond most police officers' abilities (Blaney 2010; Hirschel and Deveau 2017). My goal was to make an academic contribution to augment my professional work toward improving police response protocols to incidents of domestic violence. The intent of my doctoral study was to contribute to the academic and professional body of knowledge into police response to domestic violence. To me, this would create and establish increased credibility from a police officer with professional and academic credentials and to bridge a gap. It was my experience that there were opposing views and approaches by law enforcement, legal and judicial entities, and domestic violence protective services advocates. There was no study I was aware of that specifically studied the lived experience of police officers responding to incidents of domestic violence.

Police officers have been and continue to be maligned by women's advocacy groups, feminists, and female victims on response to domestic violence (Balenovich et al. 2008; Garner and Maxwell 2009). Some of this criticism is well deserved and some of it is not; my project was aimed to provide police with a voice. Research studies examining the perspectives of female victims of domestic violence is replete, but there are scant studies into a police officer's experience (Horwitz et al. 2011; Knowles 1996). It was my position that if I could academically present the police experience into responding to domestic violence, there could be better understanding. It was also my intention on becoming an advocate for protecting the victims of domestic violence when I retired from my police service. I wanted to be both an educator on the professional and academic side as well as a facilitator toward establishing a holistic liaison. What I was seeking was to become part of a much larger collaboration in developing discourse and consensus and reducing animus toward police. I have experienced the hostility toward law enforcement response to domestic violence by a variety of criminal justice professionals and advocacy groups. On the same token, I have also experienced the positive responses from victims I have helped, and women and children I have rescued.

I have also received accolades, awards, and recognition for my work in domestic violence intervention and prevention from victim advocate and women's groups. What I wanted to do was to translate those experiences into a positive endeavor to reduce the number of incidents of domestic violence. Unfortunately, my academic pursuit ended for a variety of reasons and I simply burned out after 16 years, with a sense of failure. I did, however, make two significant discoveries in my research into why police officers do not respond optimally to incidents of domestic violence. While I could not understand why police officers had so much difficulty determining a primary aggressor; I had made a rather astounding discovery. I discovered that police officers are only trained in the technical, structural, and legal elements of domestic violence response and nothing more. My research revealed that the use of violence in intimate relationships is fundamentally different between men and women, a gap in police training. Men use violence as a tool to intimidate and control their partners, where women used violence that did not involve these two elements (Dasgupta 2001; DeKeseredy and Dragiewicz 2007; Swan et al. 2008). While police officers cannot and should not be trained psychologists, this critical information has never been incorporated into domestic violence training in Florida (Florida Department of Law Enforcement 2022a, b).

I argued that if this is integrated into academy, field, and advanced domestic violence training, incidents of misidentifying primary aggressors would be reduced. I believed that providing line officers and supervisors with this enhanced training would lead to a more effective approach to domestic violence intervention. While my journey did not result in completing my doctorate, my hope is that this bit of information may influence a positive change. In the end, I know that there are eight women and children whose lives I made a difference in by escaping domestic violence. To the young lady that I failed, I will hopefully meet her again on the other side and apologize for my epic failure. The best compliment I received was from my mom shortly before she passed away in October 2012 and the absolution I was seeking. She told me this:

> *"I have something to tell you, your two boys, my grandsons, they have turned out to be fine young men. They are stable, responsible, well-adjusted and fine young men. You did a great job raising them and I am so proud of you, you broke the cycle."*

For me, this was absolution, because I was a terrible son to my mom and I wanted to tell her I was sorry. Unfortunately, she was too ill to have a conversation and I am hopeful that she knew how I felt prior to her passing. In the end, while my PhD journey was unsuccessful; I am happy to know that both of my sons are doing very well. I was never destined to attain the PhD, but I know that I have broken the cycle of violence in my own family.

References

Balenovich J, Grossi E, Hughes T. Toward a balanced approach: defining police roles in responding to domestic violence. Am J Crim Justice. 2008;33(1):19–31. https://doi.org/10.1007/s12103-007-9028-5.

Blaney E. Police officers' views of specialized intimate partner violence training. Policing. 2010;33(2):354–75. https://doi.org/10.1108/13639511011044939.

Collins English Dictionary. EQ. In: Collins English Dictionary—complete and unabridged. 12th ed. New York: HarperCollins; 2014. https://www.thefreedictionary.com/EQ.

Cooper FR. Who's the man? Masculinities studies, terry stops, and police training. Columbia J Gend Law. 2009;18(3):671–742. https://doi.org/10.2139/ssrn.1257183.

Dasgupta SD. Toward an understanding of women's use of non-lethal violence in intimate heterosexual relationships. Violence Against Women. 2001;8:1364–89. https://doi.org/10.1177/107780102762478046.

DeKeseredy WS, Dragiewicz M. Understanding the complexities of feminist perspectives on woman abuse. A commentary on Donald G. Dutton's Rethinking Domestic Violence. Violence Against Women. 2007;13(8):874–84. https://doi.org/10.1177/1077801207304806.

Domestic Relations. Chapter 741 marriage; domestic violence. Title XLIII § 741.29 domestic violence; investigation of incidents; notice to victims of legal rights and remedies; reporting. 2021. http://www.leg.state.fl.us/Statutes/index.cfm?App_mode=Display_Statute&Search_String=&URL=0700-0799/0741/Sections/0741.29.html.

Florida Department of Law Enforcement. Criminal justice training standards: active courses. Florida Law Enforcement Academy (Version 2021.07). Florida Department of Law Enforcement. 2022a. https://www.fdle.state.fl.us/CJSTC/Curriculum/Active-Courses.aspx.

Florida Department of Law Enforcement. Online mandatory training: domestic violence. Online mandatory training: domestic violence. 2022b. http://www.fdle.state.fl.us/FCJEI/Online-Training/Domestic-Violence.

Garner JH, Maxwell CD. Prosecution and conviction rates for intimate partner violence. Crim Justice Rev. 2009;34(1):44–79. https://doi.org/10.1177/0734016808324231.

Hirschel D. Making arrests in domestic violence cases: what police should know. Washington: U.S. Department of Justice; 2009. p. 1–2. https://www.ncjrs.gov/pdffiles1/nij/225458.pdf.

Hirschel D, Deveau L. The impact of primary aggressor laws on single versus dual arrest in incidents of intimate partner violence. Violence Against Women. 2017;23(10):1–22. https://doi.org/10.1177/1077801216657898.

Horwitz SH, Mitchell D, LaRussa-Trott M, Santiago L, Pearson J, Skiff DM, Cerulli C. An inside view of police officers' experience with domestic violence. J Fam Violence. 2011;26(8):617–25. https://doi.org/10.1007/s10896-011-9396-y.

Knowles J. Police culture and the handling of domestic violence: an urban/rural comparison. Canberra: Criminology Research Council; 1996. p. 1–252. http://www.criminologyresearch-council.gov.au/reports/41-93-4.pdf.

Lake Mary Police Department. Domestic or dating violence. Lake Mary: Lake Mary Police Department; 2018.

Prokos A, Padavic I. 'There oughtta be a law against bitches': masculinity lessons in police academy training. Gend Work Organ. 2002;9(4):439–52. https://doi.org/10.1111/1468-0432.00168.

Swan SC, Gambone LJ, Caldwell JE, Sullivan TP, Snow DL. A review of research on women's use of violence with male intimate partners. Violence Vict. 2008;23(3):301–14. https://doi.org/10.1891/0886-6708.23.3.301.

Thurman v. City of Torrington. Civ. No. H-84-120 (505 F. Supp. 1521 DC D. Conn 1984). 1984. https://www.courtlistener.com/opinion/1683702/thurman-v-city-of-torrington/.

Workman B. 'Casing the joint': explorations by the insider-researcher preparing for work-based projects. J Work Learn. 2007;19(3):146–60. https://doi.org/10.1108/13665620710735356.

Rach's Endometriosis Story

Rachel Vagg and Selena Firmin

Abstract Endometriosis occurs when tissue similar to the uterine lining grows outside the uterus, causing pelvic pain and fertility issues. This surprisingly common condition started for Rachel with her first period, in primary school, but was not diagnosed for many years. Her journey into research into this debilitating condition has just begun.

Keyword Endometriosis

1 Introduction

Period, also called menstruation, is a natural bleeding that occurs once a month as part of a woman's fertility cycle. Each month, the inside layer of the uterus thickens to prepare for a possible pregnancy. When no pregnancy occurs, the inside layer breaks down and emanates from the woman's body (Department of Health and Aged Care 2023). Endometriosis occurs when tissue similar to the uterine lining grows outside the uterus, causing pelvic pain and fertility issues. It can start during a woman's first period and last until menopause. In Australia, over 830,000 (more than 14%) girls and women deal with endometriosis at some point in their lives, usually starting in their teenage years (Endometriosis Metriosis Australia 2023). This is Rach's story of her struggle to get healthcare professionals to diagnose and treat her for endometriosis.

R. Vagg
Centre for Smart Analytics, Federation University, Mt. Helen, VIC, Australia

S. Firmin (✉)
Institute of Innovation, Science and Sustainability, Federation University, Ballarat, VIC, Australia
e-mail: s.firmin@federation.edu.au

A. Stranieri et al. (eds.), *Research Partners with Lived Experience*,
https://doi.org/10.1007/978-981-97-0033-2_10

2 Diagnosis

I got my first period when I was 11, in year six of primary school. I was the first of my friends to get it, although my cousin, 4 months younger than me, had also experienced her first period early. Very few girls had gotten their period when I got to high school. No one talked about who had their period and who did not. Different adults at the school did not treat me compassionately, so it did not surprise me that no one talked about it. My pain was brushed off multiple times by female staff members. One instance in year 7 happened when I was sitting in class crying. The teacher pulled me out of class. She seemed very frustrated with me and asked what was wrong. I told her I had my period, and she sent me to sick bay. I was still crying from the pain and humiliation of crying in front of my peers. The office lady again asked me what was wrong. I said I had my period, and I was in pain. She replied "oh you just have cramps". This annoyed me. I didn't know the pain should not have been as bad as it was. It was distressing that adult women who were supposed to nurture and support me, brushed me off so casually. I got my dad to pick me up from school that day. After that, if I thought the pain would be bad, my mum suggested I have the day off, which I greatly appreciated.

The extreme pain every month continued for a few years until I was prescribed the contraceptive pill, Levlen ED, at age 16 by my local general practitioner. Levlen ED can make a woman's periods lighter and more regular, easing period pain (Monthly Index of Medical Specialities 2020). I now know that this was the wrong pill for me. The side effects include acne, stomach pain, changes in weight, headaches, mood changes, depression, and more. Levlen ED did not even stop my cramping. I became depressed and contributed to an aversion to school. Secondary school was tough for me mentally. I hated school. Spending 7 hours a day in an environment I didn't like was draining as well as taking extra hormones that negatively impacted my way of thinking. I wish the doctor who prescribed Levlen ED, and all the doctors I saw for the next 2 years would have known and understood me better and seen that Levlen ED was not a good fit for me.

When I was 18, I decided to try an Implanon. This small plastic tube was placed under the skin in my upper arm and slowly released progesterone into my bloodstream. The Implanon can last up to 3 years and is deemed very effective in contraception by medical health professionals (Heath Direct 2023b). After I got the Implanon my pain got worse. Until then, I still had a period every month, but they were painful. As time went on, the pain got worse and worse. I then also started to experience pain during intercourse. My general practitioner (GP) diagnosed constipation, which I knew was wrong. I felt I was not being listened to or taken seriously by the doctor.

The following year, I was experiencing many more symptoms. Not only was I still having painful periods and pain during intercourse, but I also had bloating, back pain, alternating constipation and diarrhoea, fatigue, pimples, discharge, blood clots during my period, and a constant cold for most of the winter. Acupuncture helped.

A new GP thought I might have had irritable bowel syndrome (IBS) and referred me for a colonoscopy. The gastroenterologist concluded that my bowels were completely normal. After the colonoscopy results returned normal, my GP finally referred me to a gynaecologist. The first gynaecologist suspected endometriosis and performed my first laparoscopy to remove uterine tissue outside the uterus. I later discovered that not all the tissue was removed. The protocol for a laparoscopy was to stay overnight in the hospital but under pressure from my then boyfriend and against doctor's orders, I left. This was a mistake. For a couple of weeks, I continued to bleed. The gynaecologist put me on tranexamic acid briefly to stop the bleeding. This worked, and all of my symptoms subsided for a few months. Then I went back to what I considered my normal. It took many months and another gynaecologist to perform a second surgery that found more endometriosis in difficult to reach areas. He implanted an intrauterine device (IUD), a small device placed in the uterus to prevent pregnancy and can work effectively for at least 5 years (Heath Direct 2023a).

Although I had an IUD I continued to bleed, and my gynaecologist prescribed the contraceptive pill Femme-Tab ED, a type of birth control pill. The active pills contain two different female hormones in small amounts (Monthly Index of Medical Specialities 2017). Although this pill worked for quite a while, I started to spot randomly and started to experience pain with intercourse again, and if I ever forgot to take the pill, I would bleed and experience pain for a couple of days. After this, the gynaecologist took me off the pill and prescribed progesterone as he felt this would stop the bleeding. Right now, I am only 24 years old, and this will be a lifelong journey.

3   Endometriosis Research

I first got interested in research when I commenced university studies and completed a Bachelor of Criminal Justice. In one of my first courses, I was required to do an annotated bibliography on a topic of my choice. I chose to select papers on endometriosis. In the second year, I completed a literature review on endometriosis, and in the third year, I completed two research reports. One was on endometriosis, and the other was on chronic kidney disease (CKD). I don't know what I'll do next to do with research on endometriosis but the literature reviews over the last 3 years have helped me understand better what's happening to me, and how this impacts so heavily on so many young women. More research needs to be done on the diagnosis, treatment and cure for endometriosis. In addition, more specialised training in endometriosis is required for gynaecologists.

References

Department of Health and Aged Care. Menstruation (periods). 2023. Available https://www.healthdirect.gov.au/menstruation. Accessed 14 October.

Endometriosis Metriosis Australia. Some endometriosis facts. 2023. Available https://endometriosismetriosisaustralia.org/. Accessed 14 October.

Heath Direct. Intrauterine contraceptive device (IUD). 2023a. Available https://www.healthdirect.gov.au/intrauterine-contraceptive-device-iud. Accessed 14 October.

Heath Direct. Contraceptive implant. 2023b. Available https://www.healthdirect.gov.au/contraceptive-implant. Accessed 14 October.

Monthly Index of Medical Specialities. Femme-Tab ED 20/100. 2017. Available https://www.nps.org.au/assets/medicines/d918dac5-06a9-4699-b115-a53300ff90e8-reduced.pdf. Accessed 14 October.

Monthly Index of Medical Specialities. Levlen ED. 2020. Available https://www.nps.org.au/assets/medicines/84258206-0547-41e8-91cd-a53300fefe2f-reduced.pdf. Accessed 14 October.

A Peek into the Life of an Asthmatic

Sherin Tresa Paul

Abstract My journey as an asthmatic started even before I was conceived. The maternal family tree was rich in the Asthma genes and inhalers were stacked in the fridge like butter. This chapter is a narrative of events in my life from childhood since steroids became my best buddy, yet later in life caused me weight gain, polycystic ovarian disease (PCOD), and immense pain due to a condition called avascular necrosis (AVN) of bilateral femoral heads which led to two hip surgeries. There are several personal accounts which had to be included, without which the tale of this incapacitating illness would not be complete. Having gone under the blade twice, once for a tonsillectomy and then bilateral hip-core decompression with bone marrow aspiration for AVN, the total hip replacement (THR) was a breeze, or so I thought till the anesthesia wore off. The final pages present my post-surgical adventurous flight to Australia and university life as a PhD scholar.

Keywords Lived experiences · Asthma · Steroids · Avascular necrosis · Total hip replacement

1 Introduction

When you have a cold or a flu, the life as you know it is disrupted. However, as soon as you are cured, things go back to normal. This is not the case for a person who lives with a chronic illness, as this is an illness which lasts beyond a 6 month period (Yeo and Sawyer 2005). One of the many factors of chronic illness is the uncertainty associated with it (Landis 1996). The uncertainty leads to a state of constant fear

S. Tresa Paul (✉)
Institute of Innovation, Science and Sustainability, Federation University,
Melbourne, VIC, Australia
e-mail: spaul@students.federation.edu.au

© The Author(s), under exclusive license to Springer Nature Singapore Pte
Ltd. 2024
A. Stranieri et al. (eds.), *Research Partners with Lived Experience*,
https://doi.org/10.1007/978-981-97-0033-2_11

135

and my life became a tale of guarded moments. When chronic illness comes up in early childhood, the implications are much more severe. I hope that the following narrative would help the health research community to have an insight into the life of the people who struggle with early onset asthma.

2   Childhood or Something Like it

My wonderful childhood memories are tainted with the rushed nightly visits to the emergency department (ED) with my dad in tow. As soon as seeing me getting attended by the doctor and safely in a hospital bed, my dad would go to the doctor to check his blood pressure. The rest of the hospital visit would be filled with my attempts to make my dad smile by secretly making faces at the nurse who was busily poking and prodding me with a needle on all visible veins, while making small air bubbles on my arm. Accepting defeat, she would move on to the next arm and repeat the sequence while I would try not to wince with pain in front of my dad. In my mind, the people who witnessed an asthma attack suffered more than the people who are having one. That doesn't mean it was a piece of cake though. I have watched a single child bringing down an entire ward, making havoc just for one injection. Yet, here I was, sticking out my arm with a bored expression on my face as soon as the nurse arrived at the scene. I knew that the small needle prick would bring relief after hours of struggling for breath. Usually, it's the nurse who makes small talk to distract a child, but in my case, I would be the one congratulating the nurse on his/her skills in administering an injection. I was the brave little kitten who never backed down or looked away.

The charade of hospital visits, followed by injections and nebulization was not just a nocturnal event. My teachers also have had the pleasure of accompanying me to the nearest hospital while I gasped for breath with several out of tune violins in my chest playing incessantly. I was kept away from a lot of things as my loved ones feared any of them might trigger an asthma attack. The simple joys of having an ice cream, gulping down a chilled glass of mango juice, a window seat drive with wind on my face, a bare foot walk, enjoying the rain with my friends, and even the morning drill during assembly; everything was forbidden for me. I missed many functions which were far from home. If we were traveling at all, I was sure to be dressed up like a mummified corpse. My last memory as a child on stage, participating in cultural events was in kindergarten. I received the all-rounder award and I spent that in ED clutching the gold medal which had lost its shine overnight. I have always avoided looking at that gold medal displayed in the living room showcase. For the rest of my school life, I would watch from the sidelines how everyone practiced and went on stage winning dance competitions, since it was determined that I was allergic to the make-up used for dance.

I didn't even have the chance to watch a movie in a theater until I was in college, as it was air conditioned. My airways were always on alert (I was the dust detector), and I never slept without having three pillows stacked on each other so that I can breathe easier. Now I have successfully reduced it to two pillows, but I still have a bulging bump (or a hump) on my upper back. There are several studies on the posture of people with asthma (Chaves et al. 2010), including physical activity in asthmatic children and its effect on body posture (Brzęk et al. 2019).

School trips came and went, and for obvious reasons I never got to go anywhere. During lunch breaks, when kids would play on the ground, under the sun, getting drenched in sweat and covered in dust, I would be walking under the shade of trees or sitting in the classroom with another girl who had another health condition, discussing the number of tablets we take and their colors. I know my family did the best for me under the circumstances but in a way, I was robbed of my childhood. Even though it may seem like a bleak picture, I was immensely loved, and I am grateful for that.

Growing up, I understood that having a normal childhood is very important and it makes all the difference in one's life. Getting a chance to live as a kid, free of woes would play a big part in my future. No matter how many difficulties one faces in adult life, it doesn't even come close to the impact of struggles faced as a child. There was always a shadow reminding me of the missed opportunities and simple pleasures of life. I also think it gives one a much-needed perspective to have so many hardships at such an early age, so I have no regrets for the life I have had so far. Come to think of it, I have become a bookworm owing to the lack of outdoor activities. I have always been proud of myself for being a voracious reader renowned for devouring books in just a day or two. I made sure to pass on that habit to my niece and nephews as well. My heart brims with pride seeing the glint in their eyes when I gift them a book, or while they mesmerize everyone with their dances, owning the stage. In a way I am living my childhood through them. My adolescence was more or less the repetition of my childhood, so let's skip to the next phase.

3   College Life and First Job

College life was different, and I found my rebel self, choreographing, and leading in dance competitions with my trustful inhalers in my backpack. I still was an asthmatic, still visited the ED without fail at least once every 2 months, followed by a rigorous dose of antibiotics and steroids, but I had found my joy in dance. I was living precariously. I missed most of the classes as my life was spent between falling sick, getting hospitalized, and recovering. Keeping up with others in class was becoming a humongous task. Yet somehow, I managed to get by. Yes, "getting by" was enough for me those days. Ambitions were not even in the horizon as I was merely living from one asthma attack to another.

The medical system in India is different to other countries. I had no medical insurance to cover the cost of a hospital stay or for the medications. My parents, who were working as teachers, spent so much of their hard-earned money on my

health, but never complained. Even though I had only the mental capacity of a teenager, I think I regretted my existence to some extent even in those days. There was
always a shadow of melancholy following me around. However, I learned to find
happiness from little things for I knew that those blissful moments last only for so
long. I could adapt to any situation, and I never complained. I never knew that this
aspect of my character would become my Achilles heel later in life. I realize now, I
should have asked for my share of happiness, and I shouldn't have let others do a
parade on my self-worth.

I did my bachelor's degree in information technology (IT) and so my fated job
was among computers. The air-conditioned office space, which was cool enough to
make the computers live long lives, made me sick and bedridden in no time. I was
plagued with several bouts of asthma attacks and pneumonia which dipped into my
savings. My immune system was compromised, and once, on the day of discharge
from the hospital I got chickenpox too. After recovering from the chickenpox, I
started to have seizures which I kept to myself as I didn't want my family to worry.
Ayurvedic treatment brought the migraines and seizures under control. After much
retrospection, I decided to resign from the job which crippled my health to a point
of no return. Looking back, I cannot find the logic of getting into a career path like
IT where I would be confined to air-conditioned spaces. It was the time when IT
boom was happening, and students were flocking to the courses which ensured a
job. However, it led me to where I am today, as a PhD student in Australia with a full
scholarship, so I don't regret that choice.

4   The Move to Bangalore

When I was 23 years old I got married and moved to Bangalore because my husband worked there. It is one of the worst places for an asthmatic to live. The city was
notorious for its pollution, traffic blocks, and the constant architectural developments. My asthma attacks became more frequent, and I had to be on antibiotics and
steroids almost every month. My tonsils were becoming so enlarged that I became
a subject of study among the doctors who treated me. Soon enough, I was resistant
to almost all antibiotics. The doctors said that my tonsils need to be removed and I
had my first surgery, Tonsillectomy, which came with its own complications. A few
days after the surgery, a cauterized nerve ending on the surgical site came off and a
torrential bleeding began. Fortunately, my father was there, and he took me to the
hospital as fast as he could breaking several traffic rules in the process. I never
thought I had so much blood in my body. The pungent smell of blood filled the car
as it saturated my favorite bath towel, which I sadly had to discard at the hospital.
At the hospital they kept replacing the bowl in my lap that I was throwing up blood
into. I looked like a vampire who got food poisoning. Even after two tranexamic
acid injections, the bleeding didn't stop, and I was about to be taken to the operation
theater for another procedure to locate and cauterize the bleeder. Luckily, a clot
formed, and the bleeding was controlled at the last moment.

Each hospitalization was associated with multiple doses of intravenous, oral, and inhaled steroids. The moon face and acne were yet another disturbing side effect of intensive steroid treatment. When I went to Bangalore, I was 52 kilograms (kgs) and after a few years, my weight increased to 72 kgs bringing along several other problems. I was apprehensive of going out or being photographed. My smile stopped reaching my eyes because I knew I would not look good in pictures. I didn't need yet another reminder of that. I could see myself going up the ladders of dress sizes, from medium (M) to large (L) to extra-large (XL) and to XXL.

I joined post-graduation studies in the nearby engineering college. However, the constant hospitalizations became a villain there as well. I had exceeded all my medical leave and had to drop my studies after a while. Absenteeism in asthma patients is yet another issue which has been researched by many (Dean et al. 2009; Hsu et al. 2016; Bonilla et al. 2005; Kim et al. 2020). I struggled silently in a city which was making me sicker by the day.

As if all of this was not enough, polycystic ovarian disease (PCOD) was also brought into the mix which caused more pressure. My father took upon himself the task of treating me with a Siddha Ayurvedic treatment which was quite strenuous and expensive but well-known for curing asthma. I stayed at my sister's house for the treatment while her kids helped keep my spirits up. It was an intense treatment regime and was very difficult to go through, but it helped to keep the frequent asthma attacks at bay. My weight came down to 60 kgs in a few months' time and I became pregnant.

For a little while I got to see a ray of hope. I welcomed the nausea, vomiting, and every little bothersome changes in my body with both arms. I talked to my baby in the early morning hours, touching my belly. However, I lost my child on October 17, 2015, due to undiagnosed hypothyroidism. I was using sanitary pads as the bleeding was getting severe. My baby came down and rested on the sanitary pad. I cradled the tiny body in the deafening silence of the hospital bathroom, my womb crying on my behalf. When I opened the door eventually, I was forced by the hospital staff to throw my little baby into a rubbish bin covered in black polythene. The nurse too must have been traumatized and got confused what to do in such a sensitive situation. I still feel like going back to that hospital room, taking back my child, and never letting go of my baby in that way. It was the first trimester and the baby's features were just getting developed. Hardly the size of my pinky, two little dots for eyes, tiny buds in place of limbs, two lines for lips, and a cute little head which resembled an alien who had a sharp chin, just like me. This image was imprinted onto my mind forever. I am not even getting into the ordeal at the hospital prior to the miscarriage. I was given false hope that there was a chance to get a heartbeat and several scans were done while the bleeding was getting heavier and heavier. As I was blindly believing the "expert" gynecologist's words that they are still looking for a heartbeat, I didn't want to harm my already suffering child with painkillers. The pain was intolerable, and I keeled over sometimes squinting at the door of the scanning room and praying for it to open. Even today, 8 years after the loss, I still ache for my baby on October 17. I didn't realize then that in a few more years, I would be grieving the untimely demise of my marriage too.

5   Steroids: Life Saver or Villain

All through 2015, I was having moderate to severe hip pain. It was worse at nights, and I thought it may be because of the household work in the daytime. I tried everything, literally every single pain balm, oils, and my own concoctions which I slathered from my waist down. For half an hour or so, there would be a cooling effect and I'd stack up pillows under my knees (thanks to the YouTube tips) and rested on bed till the throbbing subsided to a bearable level. The level of pain was increasing day by day and I started taking painkillers, sometimes two at a time so that I can do the household chores and cooking. Quite often, I pitied my kidneys and would try to stop taking painkillers at night and lay awake till 5–6 am in the morning in intense pain, begging the sleep to come. By 6 am though the war of health consciousness vs. pain would come to an end and I would take two painkillers and sleep.

Finally, we decided to get an X-ray and look into the persistent hip pain. The doctor looked at my X-ray for a while and said, "well, there's nothing serious, just to be on the safe side, take an MRI." The result of the magnetic resonance imaging (MRI) was not as expected though. I was diagnosed with steroid induced avascular necrosis (AVN) on both hips (stage I on the right hip and stage II on the left). We were informed that a total hip replacement (THR) is unavoidable in the future. To postpone the THR surgery, we were told to do another smaller, less invasive surgery called bilateral hip core decompression with bone marrow aspiration, so we decided to get the core decompression surgery done in Bangalore, India.

6   Getting Back Up

After the core decompression surgery, the pain didn't just magically go down and I was on more medications than before. I felt like I was on a boat with no oars, thunderstorms rolling around me, pushing and pulling me in different directions with no sight of shore. My father, always a visionary, began pushing me to do the master's degree which I left halfway, this time in a different city, staying in a hostel so that I can properly recover from the hip surgery. I didn't have the strength or confidence in me to pursue higher studies as I was quite sure that I would not be able to complete. He never gave up the pursuit and finally I relented. Even though the Siddha Ayurvedic treatment helped, I was still an asthmatic, and I had the AVN pain too. Nevertheless, I welcomed the change of scenery. My brother was teaching in the same university. I was mostly bedridden for the second year, and I managed to write three technical papers in that year while doing my project, all using a bedtable. My teachers, especially my project guide Dr. Raimond, were very supportive and appreciative of my works. This boosted my morale and has helped me get back on two feet.

There were bad days too. However, I had good friends, good food, great teachers, and a pleasant atmosphere around me which slowly but surely nudged my self-worth forward into light. Bits and pieces of my lifeless mind had started to heal and began showing signs of life. Against all odds, I came second in my batch when I graduated in 2018 and I received cash awards with my head held high for consistently scoring first or second rank in all the semesters. I thank my father for pushing me out of my comfort zone and being there for me, taking care of me as if I were a newborn. In all sense, I was indeed a newborn in mind, body, and spirit.

7 Stepping into Research

It was around this time, I got an opportunity to go to Vienna, Austria, on a research stay working as a Guest Researcher under the Computer Vision Lab, TU Wien, for a project in Ambient Assisted Living (AAL). I had a taste for research and wanted to conduct research into what I have experienced my whole life, i.e., asthma and steroids. Several questions plagued my mind that needed to be answered. After coming back from Austria, I applied for a PhD in Federation University, Australia, through my aunt, an educational consultant. I got admission with a full tuition fee scholarship as well as a Health Innovation and Transformation Centre (HITC) PhD scholarship. I was intrigued by the dearth of studies which linked the inevitable progression of an asthmatic to AVN if they are put on an enormous dose of steroids over a short period. Psychosocial aspects like absenteeism from school and the marathon to keep up with the curriculum in the limited amount of "healthy time" available to an asthmatic has also not been widely researched. The research topic of my PhD proposal, "Steroids and Avascular Necrosis: An Attempt to Improve Quality of Life Through a Digital Support System," is a chapter taken from my own life.

8 Finding Myself at Atmamitra

The raging AVN pain had returned to my life, and I had to rely on painkillers again. I had been going through hell and back. The traumatic experiences of several surgeries and the issues associated with it left numerous wounds in me. Not to mention the THR which was waiting for me in my near future. My usual venting was done during confessions and after one such confession with the whole waterworks, the priest told me to contact the number on the notice board outside the church. I took down the number and called Fr. Toby Joseph S.J who gave me the general idea about the services their center Atmamitra provides, which are certain Neuro Linguistic Programming (NLP) courses (Tosey and Mathison 2010) conducted in their campus in Kerala, India, and invited me to attend the basic NLP program. In short, this was a 4-day program for healing trauma through several NLP techniques. The NLP camp is done in such a fun and friendly way with lots of ice breaking and memory games that we all felt instantly at home. This Kerala Jesuit initiative has changed the lives of several thousand people, if not more. The atmosphere itself calms down a person as it is serene and close to nature.

After completing one basic NLP program, I went ahead and joined the next camp as well. The healing is immense as you get so many chances to vent, to grieve the loss of a loved one, and to get in touch with the inner child (and this is just the tip of the iceberg). I was free to cry till there were no more tears left. I grieved the loss of my unborn child and my dearest uncle. At my third and fourth basic NLP camp, I became a volunteer in therapy sessions for the newcomers. Borrowing Fr. Toby's words, the wounded had become the healer.

The center is run with the meagre income they receive through conducting NLP camps. Even though several NLP practitioners are conducting extremely expensive courses, Atmamitra charged only Rs. 5500 (approximately 100 AUD) for the NLP course, stay, and food for 4 days. When several people asked Fr. Toby why he is charging so little, his reply was, "this is enough for me to run this center." I believe this low fees helped the people from below-average-income households to have a chance in attending this course and healing their trauma.

I stayed in Atmamitra on and off for at least two months while I was doing a course on Peace studies conducted by XLRI, Jamshedpur (Venugopal 2010) and Kerala Jesuits, India. There was a project to be done as part of the course and mine was titled "Achieving Inner Peace through Art and Inculcating a Habit of Recycling in the Younger Generation." As part of the project, I conducted an Art camp in Atmamitra, for the people, mostly teenagers, who stayed there. Some of them were treated for games and gadget addiction while some were there to get past traumatic experiences which became a roadblock in their lives. We collected discarded bottles and cans for art and several leftover cardboard bases from the birthday cakes became the canvas for budding artists. I taught them a technique called Decoupage (Lomny 1995; Nurdin et al. 2019) and they enjoyed every minute of it. It was a great success, and I had the honor of witnessing several troubled ones enjoying the process of creating something unique. On the final day we also conducted an art exhibition which boosted the confidence of every single person who was a part of the venture including myself. The unique creations were auctioned on the last day of the NLP camps conducted in the Atmamitra campus and the money received were contributed for food and birthday cakes for the Atmamitra residents. My project was selected as one of the best projects and Dr. Singh, one of the resource personnel, invited me to the XLRI, Jamshedpur campus to give a talk for the Tribals on incorporating tribal art into recyclable products as an alternative source of income. This was a really good time in my life (although short-lived). I could not make the trip as my health deteriorated fast. This is the theme of my life, the missed opportunities, and the ones sometimes I voluntarily missed because of the knowledge of the tiresome journey I would have to take on.

9 Third Time Under the Knife

I was still plagued with the AVN pain and sitting for more than 30 mins would leave me incapacitated. I had to defer the PhD program and I tried several Ayurvedic and physiotherapy treatments for the pain. It was then that the COVID-19 started, and everything went upside down not just for me, but for the whole world. Nevertheless, my hips had no care for COVID-19 or the lockdowns. I got admitted in hospital with agonizing hip pain and a new kind of pain—pins and needles in the soles of my feet. There I got yet another diagnosis, disc bulge and nerve impingement. Apparently, what my hips and feet couldn't handle was being compensated by the spine. They suggested spinal decompression therapy. It was an expensive treatment, but it gave some relief to the pain shooting down from my legs to the soles.

Apart from the disc issues, the MRI showed that the AVN had progressed from stage I to stage II on the right hip and it was progressing from stage II to stage III on the left hip. I could never put into words, the level of pain I was going through. It affected me emotionally as well. I broke down into tears easily and was quick to anger. The pain was consuming me. It was evident that the progression of AVN was speeding up and the THR surgery which seemed somewhere faraway in the horizon came dangerously close. I was waiting for the borders to open so I can commence my PhD program in Australia, but getting a THR in Australia without family support, without medical insurance (as it was a pre-existing condition), was impractical. Therefore, the THR was planned quickly and both hips were replaced in a single surgery. Although it seemed like a good idea at that time, I regret that decision now, as my recovery was very slow and even two and half years after the surgery, I am still in pain.

The doctor whom we consulted was an expert in this field. However, the nursing staff in the hospital he practiced at were notorious for being unkind and inefficient. Waking up from the surgery in blinding pain, I realized that after a major surgery, the nursing staff mattered the most and it was a harrowing experience to say the least. I had to cry and beg for pain medication from day one and they even had a joke out of it by giving me saline solution instead of pain medication, laughing, and chuckling among themselves while I writhed in pain. I was shifted from my bed to another smaller bed several times for post-surgical tests. I was being handled like a sack of potatoes while they picked me up with the bedsheet and when I cried out in pain, they snapped at me for "making a scene." For them, I was yet another patient who had a surgery. They never asked or cared that both of my hips were replaced, and I had no way of balancing myself when they threw me around from one bed to another. The agony brought by the pain was multiplied by the humiliating comments which I dare not repeat here as it would be a black mark on my country.

Normally, people would be able to get up and take a walk with crutches on the next day but in my case, the oxygen levels went down dangerously low, and I went into hypoxia. This led to more tests and more painful bed-to-trolley transfers. I dared not even defecate till I got discharged from the hospital, fearing the process of cleaning up after. They had to extend my stay by a couple of days due to the complication brought on by hypoxia and I was put on 24-hour oxygen support. I ate very little to avoid causing a mess and being cleaned up after. It was one of the worst seven days of my life and I wished and even prayed for death those first few days.

10   The Journey to Australia

Going to another country (another continent), just a few months after a major surgery was not at all acceptable for my parents, especially my father. I could see the cogs turning in his mind reflected on his clenched jaws, his furrowed brows, the constant frown and the faraway look in his eyes contemplating different worst case scenarios such as: me struggling with the two crutches and luggage in the airport lounge, falling down, calling for help, dislocating my shiny new hips in the process, or not being able to cook my own food and feed myself when I couldn't even stand without the crutches for five minutes straight as both of my hips were replaced in a single surgery so standing or balancing on "the good leg" was not possible for me since I had no "good leg" to begin with.

Thinking back now, I had taken an impossible task upon myself, but the time was naught. Australia had finally opened its borders after a long wait, and I just had to get past the border before it closed again. Thankfully I had wheelchair assistance at the airport, which made the journey bearable. I was on several painkillers but still I was shivering and wincing in pain which sometimes brought tears in my eyes amid a crowded airport. My uncle picked me up from the airport, took care of me till my pain subsided and when I assured him that I was well enough to look after myself, he dropped me to my university accommodation.

As soon as I crossed the borders, my dad learned the magic of WhatsApp video calls and started calling me every day. I should remind you that, my 82-year-old father survived three strokes, two heart attacks, and went through an angioplasty surgery. He is the pinnacle of innocence; worrying constantly about me, my siblings, and my mother; protecting us like a shield from everything that came upon us. When his call came, I was an amazing actor. I deserve an Oscar for not showing anything that's going on in my life on my face and when it wasn't humanly possible to put up an act, I didn't pick up the call.

11   A Friend in Need is a Friend Indeed

When you are in a foreign country, your friends become your family. Whenever I find myself unable to stop the tears, I'd call my friends from the nearby accommodation, who would rush to my room to see if I'm okay and they would make sure I was smiling before they left. One such night, when they got to know that I had not eaten anything for the whole day, they took me out to a KFC drive-through and fed me. They would drop me at the hospital and wait for me in the parking lot for hours till I finish up my consultation and blood tests. Sometimes they helped me pick up my medicines from the chemist or pack and move stuff for the summer room shifting, etc. Even though they were busy, they made time to help me out. Thank you so much Ewlin Varghese, Iren Mary Shimsen, Alvina Maria Jose, Chrisa Susan Shaji, Sneha Anna George, Arun Chacko, Paulson Mathew, Ansa Johnson, and Jaswin James for your kindness and thoughtfulness.

My dear friend Melissa Tayali who had her own set of problems dealing with racism and bullying was my link to reality. She would check up on me almost every week and we had fun in our own way with pizzas and movie nights. I was able to be unapologetically real in front of her and I am indebted forever to her for accepting me as who I am. My PhD colleagues, especially Hasini Gamage cheers me on, and I am grateful for the friendship which budded from late night talks and coffee runs in the midst of the research work. Anne Julie Arulnathan, a medical student from Monash University, was yet another housemate with whom I bonded instantly. It was evident that our connection was destined, and she quickly evolved into my closest confidante and dearest friend. I am eternally thankful for these two angels residing under my roof and in my heart.

Last but not the least, I thank my friend/mentor Anita Van Rooyen, confidence coach in Australia, who cheered me on and gave me much needed hugs virtually, who sent me warm clothes and shoes to keep me from freezing in the winter. I am incredibly blessed to have such kind angels in my life, and I would never be able to thank them enough in this lifetime.

12   The Supervisor Who Became My Guardian Angel

My supervisor, Dr. Lim being there for me literally at any time of the day (or night), is a crucial part of my survival here in Australia. She became a person to whom I could open myself up to. To me, she was an anchor which won't fail or falter during the storms that wrecked me again and again. I was like a clay pot, being hammered and struck down to the floor repeatedly. Each time, I desperately searched for the shattered and scattered broken pieces, gluing them back together, one piece at a time. Sometimes the pieces were glued back in the wrong places leaving gaping holes which were so evident to the onlookers. The façade of all too perfect Sherin, who endured everything with a smile, who made everything seem so easy and doable was disappearing so fast. I was grasping at straws. The stack of cards I've built up ever so carefully has begun to lose its footing. Every time I started to crumble down, Dr. Lim was there to help me get back up and I am forever grateful for her support.

13   An Opportunity of a Lifetime

It was during this time that Dr. Foale, my principal supervisor, talked about the Call for papers (CFP) for this book chapter in our weekly review meeting. People may call it destiny, but I'd like to call it a divine intervention. I decided to go for it, even though it brought forth all my insecurities so fast that I was almost blinded by it. It was difficult to look back and to let others see what I saw. For some reason unbeknownst to me, a person living with a chronic illness is not fully accepted by the society. Writing this book chapter was a cathartic experience as I was able to look at the struggles through a looking glass. The process was painful and invigorating which yielded me several notions about the issues of people suffering from AVN that need to be addressed as well as the way it needs to be approached and executed.

14   Submitting the First Draft and the Meeting with Kaya

Dr. Lim saw the need for an unbiased and well-versed eye to look through this work. She proposed bringing along Dr. Prpic (Kaya) into the team and she graciously accepted our request. Being a pioneer in her field, I expected Kaya to grill me on the aspects of my writing, so I was ready with my journal and my favorite four colored pen. What happened was truly surprising. She let me talk about my condition and my bitter experiences while asking questions which compelled me to look into my soul and spit out the truth which no therapist who charged me $175 per hour has ever managed to do.

She cracked open my shell in a matter of minutes and all the blood and gore started to spill through the cracks, quite brazenly. Halfway through the meeting, my pen still in my hand and the journal page in front of me bare, I asked her what she felt about my writing. She was quite straightforward and told me the truth that I was narrating the "events" happened in my life in a chronological order without letting others see how I experienced it. I would say, in a way she called my bluff. I have always distanced myself from the ugly reality of it all. In fact, I made fun of my illnesses to make my friends and family laugh. How could I possibly show anyone what really was happening to me? All my life I regretted my existence, so I tried my best to silence the agony and play the happy go lucky act, which I perfected over the time.

What I wrote about my childhood in my first draft ended with me getting a gold medal for being an all-rounder in my kindergarten and later being rushed to the hospital at night while I tied myself to the gold medal. She saw through it instantly and asked me "where is the rest of your childhood?". Childhood goes all the way through till teenage years and I had jumped right from that eventful night in kindergarten to college life. That must have been the longest jump in history. I realized that, from that fateful night in the kindergarten, the child in me stopped being a kid. Dancing was my passion and after being diagnosed with asthma, I was not allowed to dance, as the doctor concluded that the make-up used in the dance caused my allergic reaction. Since then, I was kept away from all strenuous physical activities. Kaya advised me to write and express myself as though I am dancing. I went back and started to peel off the scar tissues which covered my childhood memories.

15 Panic Attacks and the Little Victories

A review on post-traumatic stress disorder (PTSD) after surgeries sheds light on the post-surgical struggles a person might endure (El-Gabalawy et al. 2019). This paper discusses the intraoperative awareness and its correlation to PTSD. I distinctly remember hearing my artificial hips being hammered into place, and the unnatural metallic sound in the operation theater still brings me chills. It felt like an hour of intermittent hammering sounds while they turned me and repeated the same procedure on both hips. I remember feeling breathless the whole time. It was unlike the breathlessness of asthma. It felt like someone was choking me, and no matter how deep I breathed, there was no air entering my body. It seemed like I was on the brink of death. Yet, I'd say, the post-operative "nursing care" I received was more traumatic than this unfortunate experience of intraoperative awareness.

After the THR surgery, I've been having panic attacks. This followed me to Australia too. I tried everything to stop the hammering in my chest and the impending doom from swallowing me up. Here's a free advice: never search Google or YouTube for ways to stop a panic attack while you are having one. There was no proper rehabilitation after the THR surgery and in a new country with such pain and uncertainty, I struggled every single day for even the simple tasks of cooking, cleaning, or having a shower. Sometimes, I looked at the random things which I couldn't pick up from the floor and I hated myself for it with passion. After a while though, I managed to pick up things from the floor using my right leg. The left one is still on the mend. For a long time, I longed to sleep on my side. The joy I felt when I was able to sleep on my side without pain, several months after the surgery is incomparable. I would still need at least one revision surgery in 10–15 years depending upon the wear and tear and I dread the revision surgery and the recovery phase.

My routine was all over the place. Sometimes I had my breakfast at 3 pm and from time-to-time, breakfast, lunch, and dinner were packed into a single meal which I had at night when the least number of people were in the kitchen. I think this started as a way to avoid the pitiful looks I got as I walked with crutches. When my mood was low (which was quite often), I ate chocolates, lots, and lots of it. A year after the surgery, I had high cholesterol and another orthopedic condition called heterotopic ossification (HO) (Zhu et al. 2015; Zran et al. 2022) which is a serious complication of THR where islands of bone formation happen in soft tissues. This has only one viable treatment option, a revision arthroplasty (Łęgosz et al. 2019), which might affect the success rate of the joint(s) that have been replaced, not to mention the trauma associated with yet another surgery and the painful recovery phase. I still have pain, inflammation, and problems with range of motion. I will be going for my next CT and Bone Scan soon to get a clearer picture on the progression and what can be done to make the situation a bit more bearable. The prevention of HO is still a gray area wherein there are two viable options: Nonsteroidal anti-inflammatory drugs (NSAIDs) and radiation, neither of which were given to me. Among the two, radiation is said to be more effective (Cai et al. 2019).

16   Some Pearls of Wisdom I Picked Up on the Way

Make hay while the sun shines: make the most of the good days, be kind to yourself and accept the bad days. Find little pocketsful of happiness and hold on to it.

Pain is a symptom, do not try to numb it temporarily. It is a way your body communicates with you. Listen to it, let it show what is the underlying issue.

Do regular health check-ups, even if everything is sailing smoothly.

Be kind to others. You don't know what's the size of the stone which is stuck in their shoes. Believe me, everyone has at least one.

17   Conclusion

Even people without asthma but had undergone intensive corticosteroid treatments for COVID-19 are having AVN and THR's these days (Agarwala et al. 2021; Banerjee et al. 2021; Ergözen and Kaya 2021; Joshi et al. 2021; Sulewski et al. 2021; Zhang et al. 2021; Annam et al. 2022; Asilova and Mirzayev 2022; Mañón et al. 2022; Nurulloyev 2022; Sherikar et al. 2022; Tewatia and Singh 2022; Torgashin and Rodionova 2022). I came upon this new trend recently and though it might not come under the scope of my PhD work, I'd like to delve deep on it after completing the PhD. If not countered proactively, this would bring forth a range of repercussions like an overloaded healthcare system with unplanned THR and core-decompression surgeries, post-surgical trauma, financial struggles, care-giver's burden, dependency on pain medication, deteriorating mental health, and the lack of an effective support system. I would like to make it known to the unsuspecting global community about this avalanche waiting to happen and help them from getting lost in it. Everyone deserves to live a normal life and experience the joy that little things bring. I am hopeful that my research will bring an awareness in patients, caregivers, and healthcare professionals so that this disastrous trajectory of life in pain can be avoided.

After the PhD, I would like to teach, research, and reach young minds, train them to look for the issues people suffer through silently and make sustainable solutions for them. It wasn't easy living in a new country, while juggling with so many challenges. I am grateful for the support I received from my PhD supervisors, my friends, and Federation University, Australia for helping me through this tough time.

Acknowledgment I thank the almighty God for making me worthy enough and strong enough to bear the struggles in my life without which I never would have reached here today. I express my heartfelt gratitude to my supervisors Dr. Madhu Chetty, Dr. Cameron Foale, Dr. Suryani Lim, and Dr. Britt Klein who supported my PhD candidature in all possible ways till date. I thank the FedLiving staff, especially Ms. Marissa Pacunskis, who was really kind to me, bringing over my mails and parcels to my accommodation as it was difficult for me to walk to the campus. Thank you, Dr. Juliana Kaya Prpic, Indigenous Engineering Education Specialist, The University of Melbourne, for asking difficult questions which needed to be asked, for making me look back for the answers in the deepest darkest corners of my mind, for helping me tell my story, and for proof reading, the most tedious task.

I am thankful for the disability officer Ms. Naomi Floyd for all the help when I first arrived at the campus and for arranging me a room with an attached bathroom in the University campus. Thank you, Ms. Carly Tulloch, student support officer, for checking on me from time to time.

The guidance I received from Dr. Kumudha Raimond, who was my project guide in Karunya Institute of Technology and Sciences from where I completed the Post-Graduate degree, ignited the fire which is still burning in me today. This section would not be complete without thanking her and several other teachers who taught, supported, and helped me without expecting anything in return.

I thank my siblings Dr. Sonia Raju and Bobby P. Paul, for taking care of me when I couldn't. I am grateful for my little niece Sonam who is not so little anymore and my nephews Pavan and Gazal for lighting up my world with laughter and love.

I'm deeply thankful for my uncle Thomas Mathew and aunt Treesa Mathew, who provided invaluable support during my initial days in Australia when I arrived on a wheelchair, experiencing severe pain. They were my much-needed pitstop and lifeline during that challenging time.

If I am sitting here today and writing this acknowledgment with an unfaltering smile on my face, it is only because of the sacrifices, guidance, and prayers of my parents, Prof. P. Paul, and Catherine Paul. No words can ever suffice to thank them, so I will do my best to make them proud through my research work and in being a kind human being just as they are.

References

Agarwala SR, Vijayvargiya M, Pandey P. Avascular necrosis as a part of "long COVID-19". BMJ Case Rep. 2021;14(7):e242101.

Annam P, et al. Corticosteroids induced avascular necrosis of hip, a "long COVID-19" complication: case report. Ann Med Surg. 2022;82:104753.

Asilova SU, Mirzayev AB. Post-covid avascular necrosis of the femoral head. Web Scientist Int Sci Res J. 2022;3(8):228–33.

Banerjee I, Robinson J, Sathian B. Corticosteroid induced avascular necrosis and COVID-19: the drug dilemma. Nepal J Epidemiol. 2021;11(3):1049.

Bonilla S, et al. School absenteeism in children with asthma in a Los Angeles inner city school. J Pediatr. 2005;147(6):802–6.

Brzęk A, et al. Body posture and physical activity in children diagnosed with asthma and allergies symptoms: a report from randomized observational studies. Medicine. 2019;98(7):e14449.

Cai L, et al. Optimal strategies for the prevention of heterotopic ossification after total hip arthroplasty: a network meta-analysis. Int J Surg. 2019;62:74–85.

Chaves TC, et al. Craniocervical posture and hyoid bone position in children with mild and moderate asthma and mouth breathing. Int J Pediatr Otorhinolaryngol. 2010;74(9):1021–7.

Dean BB, et al. The impact of uncontrolled asthma on absenteeism and health-related quality of life. J Asthma. 2009;46(9):861–6.

El-Gabalawy R, et al. Post-traumatic stress in the postoperative period: current status and future directions. Can J Anesth. 2019;66(11):1385–95.

Ergözen S, Kaya E. Avascular necrosis due to corticosteroid therapy in covid-19 as a syndemic. Central Asian J Med Hypotheses Ethics. 2021;2(2):91–5.

Hsu J, et al. Asthma-related school absenteeism, morbidity, and modifiable factors. Am J Prev Med. 2016;51(1):23–32.

Joshi SR, et al. Post COVID-19 osteoporosis and avascular necrosis of femoral head: a case report. Int J Orthopaed. 2021;7(4):177–9.

Kim CH, Gee KA, Byrd RS. Excessive absenteeism due to asthma in California elementary schoolchildren. Acad Pediatr. 2020;20(7):950–7.

Landis BJ. Uncertainty, spiritual well-being, and psychosocial adjustment to chronic illness. Issues Ment Health Nurs. 1996;17(3):217–31.

Łęgosz P, et al. Heterotopic ossification: a challenging complication of total hip arthroplasty: risk factors, diagnosis, prophylaxis, and treatment. Biomed Res Int. 2019;2019:3860142.

Lomny A. Art of decoupage. Craft Arts Int. 1995;35:71–5.

Mañón VA, et al. COVID-associated avascular necrosis of the maxilla-a rare, new side effect of COVID-19. J Oral Maxillofac Surg. 2022;80(7):1254–9.

Nurdin N, et al. Decoupage art therapy as an alternative activity to reduce gadget dependence on primary school students in makassar [Seni Decoupage Sebagai Kegiatan Alternatif Mengurangi Ketergantungan Gadget Pada Siswa Sekolah Dasar di Makassar]. Proc Commun Dev. 2019;2:872–83.

Nurulloyev SO. Comparative characteristics of the frequency of aceptic necrosis of the femoral head after covid-19. Web Scientist Int Sci Res J. 2022;3(7):257–63.

Sherikar A, et al. Fear of avascular necrosis in COVID survivors is real: a rare case series. Eur J Mol Clin Med. 2022;9(2):1249–52. Available https://ejmcm.com/article_17754.html.

Sulewski A, et al. Avascular necrosis bone complication after active COVID-19 infection: preliminary results. Medicina. 2021;57(12):1311. https://doi.org/10.3390/medicina57121311.

Tewatia P, Singh YP. Avascular necrosis-A complication of COVID-19 infection treatment. Indian J Rheumatol. 2022;17(4):440.

Torgashin AN, Rodionova SS. Osteonecrosis in patients recovering from COVID-19: mechanisms, diagnosis, and treatment at early-stage disease. Traumatol Orthoped Russia. 2022;28(1):128–37.

Tosey P, Mathison J. Neuro-linguistic programming as an innovation in education and teaching. Innov Educ Teach Int. 2010;47(3):317–26.

Venugopal P. XLRI: "renewing the face of the earth". In: Ethics, business and society: managing responsibly. London: Sage; 2010. p. 75.

Yeo M, Sawyer S. Chronic illness and disability. BMJ. 2005;330(7493):721–3.

Zhang S, et al. Beware of steroid-induced avascular necrosis of the femoral head in the treatment of COVID-19—experience and lessons from the SARS epidemic. Drug Des Devel Ther. 2021;15:983–95.

Zhu Y, et al. Incidence and risk factors for heterotopic ossification after total hip arthroplasty: a meta-analysis. Arch Orthop Trauma Surg. 2015;135:1307–14.

Zran N, et al. Heterotopic ossification after total hip arthroplasty: radiological comparison between a direct anterior approach without an orthopaedic table and a posterior approach. Hip Int. 2022;32(5):604–9.

You Have to Be Courageous

Jet van der Voet and Tineke Abma

Abstract Leukaemia brought my son's (Pim) and our family life to a standstill. The hospital world took over our everyday life, and we had to adapt. This all had a great social-emotional impact on the whole family. It was only after Pim's death that I started working as an expert-by-experience for a better treatment of future patients. That was after I wrote a book entitled 'Superbro'. Tineke Abma asked me to become a patient-research partner in a Participatory Action Research (PAR) project in the hospital. The aim was to improve patient care through a dialogical learning process among patients, family members, nurses and doctors. This led to a collaboration with the department where my son had been treated. Along the way I learned it is important to be courageous in a context where professionals typically respond with technical solutions to fix problems. As a result, my family and many other families felt on their own to grief and mourn about what was lost and could not be repaired. In the PAR project we created a safe space to share these experiences with nurses and doctors. One of the best experiences was when I heard from other patients that things had improved at the hospital.

Keywords Dialogue · Participatory action research · Experiences · Existential

1 Introduction

In this chapter I, Jet van der Voet, mother of Pim who died of leukaemia, describe my journey as a mother who became a Research Partner. From a first-person stance I share my experiences with the illness of my son and the hospital admission. The chapter is structured as follows: I start describing the overwhelming

J. van der Voet (✉) · T. Abma
Leiden University Medical Centre, Leiden, The Netherlands

A. Stranieri et al. (eds.), *Research Partners with Lived Experience*,
https://doi.org/10.1007/978-981-97-0033-2_12

151

experience of my son being seriously ill and the admission to the academic hospital. I go on to present my motivation to become a 'researcher', from who I experienced support and what lessons I have learned. I got to know Tineke Abma who approached me for a Participatory Action Research project she initiated in the hospital where my son Pim was treated. At the end of the chapter Tineke reflects on my narrative.

2   Illness Experience

My son Pim was diagnosed with leukaemia on 20 March 2018. The news came as a 'hammer blow,' as Pim himself stated it. Life as he knew it came to a standstill. No more studying. No more working. No more sport or partying. Instead, what followed was a year of hope and fear, of extremely complex and exhausting treatment which eventually proved too much for him to bear. When the disease returned a year later, and he became paralyzed, he requested euthanasia. He died on 16 May 2019 at the age of 22.

2.1   Hell and Torture

In the year of Pim's illness, we—Pim and his family—went through a lot. It felt like we had seen the hospital inside and out. Because of his illness, treatment and a long list of complications, Pim was admitted to the nursing wards of the haematology, neurology, oncology, short-stay and medium care departments. He was treated, supervised, helped, seen or referred by anaesthetists, pharmacists, dieticians, physiotherapists, gynaecologists, cardiologists, internists, dermatologists, internal medicine physicians, ear, nose and throat specialists, lung disease specialists, social workers, gastroenterologists (stomach, intestine and liver), psychiatrists, the pain centre, the accident and emergency department, radiologists, the rehabilitation centre and the urology department. The haematology polyclinic and nursing ward were his main station. Pim hated being there so much that he called the hospital 'hell' and his treatments 'tortures,' although he took it very bravely.

> His heart does not beat faster and his blood pressure does not rise, whatever the treatment. He cooperates with everything. He agrees to scans and radiation. He does not shrink from the numerous occasions when an IV tube has to be inserted or blood has to be taken. He bites back the pain during the hated epidurals and the bone marrow punctures. He suffers the side-effects, the complaints and the complications of the chemotherapy and the drugs. He is strong, stronger than the rest of us together. (Superbro, p. 31)

2.2   Losing Control

But the 'hell' that Pim alluded was not only because of the severe treatments. It was unbearable for Pim that his life has been taken from him and that he was losing grip. In the hospital, he could not live his own life anymore. His sleep was interrupted all the time, the food was miserable, his friends were not welcome. He missed his daily sport and exercise. He wanted to play his games, sitting up straight, but the table was too short to overlook the whole screen—the room was dominated by the bed. From day one he was completely absorbed in the schedule of doctors and nurses. He was effectively immobilized. His main job was to adapt and obey, sit and wait, not knowing what the next step is. He no longer had any control over his life.

The hospital paid little attention to the social and emotional aspects of the illness and the treatments. In general, doctors and nurses concentrate at their routine and have no time to really see, listen and talk to their patients. Empathy is a rare trait to be experienced or witnessed. We learn that the staff were educated to behave professionally. In hospital terms, 'professional' means 'with distance'—the opposite of the patient's need. For Pim the whole situation was so horrible—so much so that later in his journey he was diagnosed with *trauma*. In retrospect, I recognize all the phases that he suffered through during this trauma: fight, freeze and flight.

> Fighting is familiar, it is Pim's preferred strategy. During the first stage of the treatment Pim fought for all he was worth and only very occasionally displayed signs of choosing flight. Generally he bore the terrible chemotherapy like a soldier and after each session he pulled himself together and battled on. But now, after the stem cell transplant, Pim is frozen. It is pointless fighting what he is facing now. Flight is impossible. Freezing is all that is left: Pim is in survival mode. (Superbro, p.68)

2.3   Living in a Daze

But Pim was not the only one who is finding it difficult. We were also distressed: his parents, his brother and sister, family, friends. Our lives had also changed irrevocably. We tried to go on as best we could, but the concerns about Pim were always at the front of our minds. We cleared our diaries. What followed was a year without any holidays or social life, neglected housekeeping, falling behind with the bills and mechanically going through the motions at work.

> Pim's illness takes over our lives completely. Nothing else matters. We want just one thing: Pim's recovery. […] We are living in a daze, getting by on adrenaline alone. We are constantly worried. I am fearful all the time, deeply scared of losing Pim. That is the other side of the unconditional love I feel for him. Being willing to die for someone else is no longer an abstract concept. How simple the choice would be, if only it were possible. (Superbro, p. 30–31)

3   Motivation to Become a 'Researcher'

3.1   Lack of Information

During the illness and treatment of my son, I at first was hardly able to represent him. We tried to understand the situation that we were in: the leukaemia, the treatment, the medicines, the protocols, the building, the staff, the hospital life, the do's and the don'ts—everything was so very overwhelming.

After the first shock, we began to ask a lot of questions. But we did not get much of an answer. It was imposed upon us that Pim must take things one step at a time, and not look too far ahead. Taking things as they come was not one of Pim's strengths, or mine for that matter. The strong advice was not to look up information at the internet—but of course we do, and of course we only understand half of it.

> Pim's lymphoma has meanwhile been officially diagnosed as T-cell lymphoblastic lymphoma. The disease is treated as acute lymphatic leukaemia. This is new to us and we don't understand what it means. There is undoubtedly a medical plan, but we haven't a clue what awaits Pim and ourselves in the coming days, weeks and months. Nor does it become any clearer to us when the haematologist on duty walks into the room a few hours later. The doctor sits on the table, casually swinging his legs. He is wearing a lab coat, but underneath is a shirt with a floral print and cool shoes. He impresses on us that we are in a teaching hospital and stresses that Pim could be of help with academic research. He leaves behind two forms with which Pim can (must?) consent to participate in research. (Superbro, p. 18–19)

3.2   Victim and Observant

The lack of information and the unanswered questions remained a red line in the year of treatment. But there were more reasons why every day was a struggle for us. There were a lot of things that we wondered about apart from the treatment. From trivial things, like the illogical signage in the building and the old-fashioned 'line up' of students gathering around the hospital bed, to important things, such as the lack of cooperation between departments and the impossibility to get enough sleep, healthy food or exercise. And why was the staff so cold and distant? What kept them addressing Pim as 'Mr Mellink'?

Educated as an academic and a policy advisor, though in a very different field, I am used to processing a lot of information and to detect 'system errors'. In the hospital, I could not help myself doing 'research'. I was both a victim and an observer at the same time. I did not interfere in medical matters; it's the organization and financing of the hospital, the culture and habits, the hierarchy and protocols, the lack of patient perspective and participation that puzzled me. The hospital system appeared to be more of a bureaucracy to me then my own ministry. It was money-driven, focused on efficiency, research and results—not focused on patients. Sometimes I had a moment to 'interview' a nurse or a doctor—on why they were doing what they were doing? '*It's protocol*', was the most heard answer or simply '*I do as I'm ordered to*'.

> It is incomprehensible, for example, that the women who bring around refreshments knock on the door at least six times every day—even when Pim is being fed intravenously and is therefore not eating. The instructions come from above and must be followed. The women can't just skip Pim's room at their own discretion. It drives Pim mad. (Superbro, p. 71–72)

We tried very hard to adjust to the hospital manners. I tried not to complain too often. It was the same experience that I had encountered as a parent interacting with a school: as a mother, you don't criticize the teacher—it might have negative consequences for your child. But Pim himself often and openly showed and expressed his displeasure, and sometimes lost his temper. It was during those moments that I realized how courageous he was, in addressing topics that we or other patients and their families did not dare to mention. And he was not rewarded doing so.

> The Belgian ward doctor has returned specially to discuss the incident. She did not appreciate the tone Pim had adopted the previous day. 'That is not how we treat one another', she wants to tell him. I don't know precisely what Pim had said, but he made no secret of his displeasure with the way things were done in the hospital. He is very upset that the doctors are unable to find a way to relieve his pain. He also feels that the doctors show too little empathy. 'They should try lying in this bed once', he often remarks. (Superbro, p. 26)

Pim's courage grew every day. After some time, he started asking questions and making comments himself.

> For one of Pim's last visits to the hospital, we ask to meet the specialist nurse, the neurologist and the haematologist. It is 19 April 2019 and Pim wants a clear and honest appraisal of his chances. 'I have now been given T cells', he says. 'But what if they don't work?' The haematologist replies that Pim could then be given an extra dose of T cells. 'And if that still doesn't work?', Pim persists. The haematologist hesitates. 'I think we would then consider another total body irradiation'. Pim notes the hesitation: 'But if that was a good idea, wouldn't you be doing it immediately?' (Superbro, p. 115)

Where a year ago there was a large teenager sitting in the consultation room who let his parents to do the talking, there was then an adult who allowed his parents to listen in. I suddenly realized how much Pim had grown as a person and an adult. His questions were to the point, and he choose his words carefully. He was calm and he was wise. He was taking charge.

3.3   After-Care Conversation

During Pim's hospital stay I had the opportunity to see, hear, feel and think a lot. Sometimes there was a moment to wonder, but often the time in the hospital was so stressful and so much was happening, that there was no room for reflection. Real moments of reflection and evaluation came later, after Pim's death, at home, during dialogue with my family, but also in conversation with the hospital.

The first conversation we had in the hospital after Pim's death was planned as 'after-care'. We had the opportunity to ask the questions that really keep us awake at night with ponder.

> The conversation begins uncomfortably. I see the unease on the other side of the table—perhaps they are afraid that we're going to cause problems or become emotional. What we want to know it the precise cause of Pim's death: the disease or the treatment. We wonder why the cause of death was not investigated. Was that something we had to request ourselves? But isn't the LUMC an academic hospital? And why does the LUMC follow protocol so strictly? Why was Pim not given the T-cells sooner, when it was immediately apparent after the stem cell transplant that there were still cancer cells in his spinal cord? In hindsight, would the doctors have followed a different course of treatment? (Superbro, p. 175)

Of course, I knew that we would not get all the answers, although we stressed that we went in the meeting with an open mind, and we were not looking to hold the hospital liable for any malpractice. We only wanted to know more about Pim. But I saw no willingness to open up from other side. I assumed that hospital culture was dominated too much by the fear of potential legal actions and claims for damages from patients. Later, and off the record, Pim's haematologist confirmed that they really had no answers. I might have gotten paranoid by previous experiences.

3.4   Letter of No Difference

During the after-care conversation, we suggested that we would write a letter to the hospital with a family reflection on different topics. The doctors told us to write to the service centre. And so, we did: I wrote a long letter about our journey through Pim's hospital experiences. I felt the urge to do so. It felt too easy to just back off, forget all and to get back into the routine of our regular lives. I did it for Pim and for ourselves, but mainly for the other patients—'future Pims'. We had experienced more of the hospital than a regular patient, and maybe more than most associated doctors or nurses. We were effectively professional clients. In the letter, I raised a number of matters: the lack of coordination from within the hospital ('island hopping without a tour operator'); the artificial division between the polyclinic and the haematology nursing ward (which meant that Pim had no fixed haematologist); the mandatory, time-consuming intake procedure in the Accident and Emergency department where Pim had to go when any event occurred between appointments; the lack of communication between the hospital and external services; and the poor basic care which meant that Pim always 'came home dirty, hungry, and above all, very tired'. I also raised the absence of the human dimension in the Leiden University Medical Centre (LUMC) and the concern that professionalism does not necessarily require staff to be cold and distant from patients. I finally suggested that the hospital should establish a youth department as a follow-up to the children's ward.

> I don't believe that anything will actually be done with the letter. I expect the hospital to be rigid and bureaucratic. It will undoubtedly take weeks before the letter finds its way onto the right desk. I am therefore greatly surprised when just a few days later, and on a Sunday

evening, we receive an initial reaction from the LUMC's head of Medical Affairs. In the reply, we are thanked for our letter and invited to a meeting. 'I would like to thank you for this letter. For the fact that, despite your grief, you took this step. And have given us the chance to learn from his and your experiences on the basis of the journey Pim was forced to take through our house. I do not read it as an accusation, but a request to us to take a close look at ourselves in the mirror. And what we see, is that we still have a lot to do'. (Superbro, p. 182)

This nice response to my letter was followed by a meeting with the head of the service centre. The meeting helped in the sense that we felt that we had finally been seen and heard. At the same time, we had the feeling that this one letter would make no difference.

3.5   Book and Follow-Up

In honour of my son, after his death I wrote the book 'Superbro' (Van der Voet 2020). This book recorded my memories of the year during Pim's illness and was written mostly during the first national corona virus lockdown (2020). I had written it in the first place in loving memory of Pim and in proud recollection of the courage he showed while facing up to the treatment he underwent and his brave decision to end his own life (euthanasia). But also, to tell his family and friends more about the course of the disease that ultimately led to Pim's final decision. Few people witnessed his struggles during that final year first hand. For many, the progression of the disease and the final step came as a total shock. For myself, writing this book, although an extremely painful process, helped to give clarity to my thoughts about everything that happened during that terrible year—and above all to hold on to my memories of Pim. It in fact has helped in processing my own trauma.

Family and friends told me that the book could have another powerful purpose as well. They were shocked by the insight offered about hospital life and culture. Some of them suggested that I should present the book to the board of the hospital. At first, I doubted these suggestions as being a clever idea. I hesitated and had to gather courage. When after some weeks, I finally wrote an e-mail to the secretary of the board, and they responded quickly. To my surprise, one of the members of the board was glad to receive the book. Beforehand holding a meeting, he wanted to read the book, so he could discuss our experiences with us. And when we finally met, he indeed knew the book by heart and seemed genuinely displeased with Pim's story. He had reserved plenty of time to talk to us and my nerves quickly disappeared when I saw how open and honest he was being. He asked for ten more books to hand out to the other board members and hospital management. Afterwards, he kept me informed about next steps: his conversations with the haematology department and the blog of the chairman at the intranet informing the complete hospital staff. I am not sure what impression the book had truly made on the hospital, for I was no longer an intern now. But after the publication of the blog of the chairman, I did receive a lot of orders for the book, mainly from the region where the hospital is situated.

3.6 Participatory Action Research Project

Tineke Abma invited me to become a patient-research partner in a participatory action research (PAR) project at the Leiden University Medical Center hospital. The aim of this PAR project was to improve patient care through a dialogical learning process among patients, family members, nurses and doctors (Abma et al. 2019). PAR is a collaborative research approach that aims to heighten the personal and mutual understandings of those whose life and work is at stake. PAR researchers and co-researchers share control over the research process from the very first beginning to the disseminations of findings. In this case Tineke and her colleague Anne Stiggelbout designed a study in two phases. In the first phase of the project a group of patients, family members, nurses and doctors with illness experiences shared illness stories. In the second phase this research group invited and engaged hospital departments to jointly learn by sharing their own personal narratives.

4 Best Experience

4.1 PAR Project

Of course, the best experience for me working on this project was to hear that processes and culture at the hospital, and especially from within the haematology department had changed for the better. The board member told me about the positive changes, but I did not have the experience of them first hand. The leukaemia department did not want to meet me after the publication of 'Superbro'. I understood some staff had read the book, but it was apparently too painful for them to discuss what happened. I have not insisted, and I was not yet ready for what would be a real confrontation. I was nervous that Pim and us, his family, would be set apart as an exceptional case, and maybe accused of bad behaviour due to our actions. In this stage in life I lacked the courage.

Still, there have been moments of feedback which made me feel proud. The first is feedback from my friend Birgit after a 'mirror talk' with the head nurse of the leukaemia department, supervised by Tineke. Some time after the publication of 'Superbro', the leukaemia department contacted Tineke to join the PAR project. Superbro had been read as a critique and generated many emotions among the nurses and doctors in this department, so their willingness to learn from patients and family members came as a positive surprise. My book maybe had set something in positive motion. However, I felt that I was not the one to talk to them given the sensitivity of the professionals. After reflection I contacted my friend Birgit, who was willing to do so. Birgit and Tineke carefully prepared a series of two dialogues with the nurses and doctors of the department.

I met Birgit in the hospital as the wife of Edwin. Edwin had a different syndrome, but like Pim was having chemotherapy and a stem cell transplant. Since Edwin died, some months before Pim, Birgit had never set foot in the hospital again. But in my place, she had the courage to talk with the staff about her own experiences—and they were very similar to my own. Birgit told the nurses straight out how her husband and she panicked when they learned that the required T-cell boost was cancelled without proper communication. Their last hope had dissolved into the air, and there was hardly any time to cope with the bad news. She also told them how important her role was because her husband was surviving and could not make sense of the bodily responses on the treatment. Yet, she was hardly consulted with and spoken to during Edwin's treatments. Most of all, she felt like a passenger during the whole process, both dependent and powerless. Birgit reported to me that the head nurse was rather touched after hearing Edwin's story and Birgit's experiences and feelings. In fact, it enhanced my story about the haematology department. Hearing a similar story to my own, may have finally stopped the denial of the situation.

4.2   Changes at the Department

The second moment I felt proud, was hearing from Hanneke, the mother of Maud. Maud suffered from leukaemia and was hospitalized for the last time January 2022. I was in contact with her mother, and she reported some changes at the ward. In the morning, Maud could sleep in without being disturbed. The family could take home made food for Maud to the hospital, and in the day room the department finally placed a microwave (after Maud and her family made a scene). When Maud was still stable, she was permitted to have the weekend off and go home. Also, the hospital was replacing the alarm ringing IVs with silent ones. These are little changes, but oh so important steps to making the hospital life a little less 'hell'. Unfortunately, some weeks later Maud passed away.

My hopes for a better hospital life increased also when I heared from a former physiotherapist that all patients of the haematology department could join a programme of exercise now.[1] And again when I read on Facebook that the hospital had opened a 'chill room' for young adolescents at the oncological department—I hope this includes the haematological patients as well. Of course, this progress was not the result of my 'research' and the book alone. But I like to think that our conversations, the letter, the book and the PAR project have made a slight contribution.

---

[1] As secretary-general of The Netherlands Sports Council, I later wrote an article about (lack of) exercise in hospitals: Hoeveel beweging zit er eigenlijk in ziekenhuizen?|Nieuwsbericht|Nederlandse Sportraad (https://www.nederlandse-sportraad.nl).

5 Experienced Support

5.1 Specialist Nurse

Pim was 21 when he fell ill. His medical treatment, although experimental, was undoubtedly of a high standard. But little attention was paid to his social and emotional condition or his welfare. Outside organizations and other authorities also show little consideration with Pim. The university told him that it would be better if he stopped studying immediately, working was no longer possible, he did not qualify for a regular or disability benefit and the procedures under the Social Support Act took so long, that they would eventually be processed after Pim's death. He had only family to fall back on.

In the hospital we experienced little support whatsoever, until we met with the specialist nurse, who was carefully monitoring Pim's condition after the stem cell transplant. This specialist nurse made the time to get to know Pim and the rest of us. He treated Pim with respect and took every question seriously. We have come to have enormous respect for him.

> He takes however long is necessary for a consultation and this sometimes means there is a long queue of people waiting for an appointment in the corridor. The patients all seem to accept this, since once inside he gives all of them the attention they need. Whatever the situation, the nurse conveys an enormous sense of calm. (Superbro, p. 81)

In a short time the specialist nurse was organizing everything for us: he arranged appointments with other departments which saved us a huge amount of work, organized treatments, informed us of the results of tests and faxed prescriptions for pills to our own pharmacy (or to the nearest hospital if it is the evening) so that we didn't have to drive up and down from The Hague to Leiden every time. If Pim could not be reached, the nurse called Pim's father or myself. 'And how are *you* doing?', he always asked at the end of each call. It was clear that the support shown from this specialist nurse had something to do with his position, being an intermediator between patients and doctors, and between the haematology polyclinic and other departments. But he was for sure the right man in the right place. Unfortunately, he was out of the picture when Pim was staying at the haematology nursing ward—his position was tied to the polyclinic only.

5.2 Fellow Sufferers

In the hospital, we got to know some of the other patients. Their illnesses created a bond between them. Family and friends are of course very important to Pim, but as he said, they didn't really know how it is to be so very sick and face death. I feel the same way: no one can know or feel how scared I am too loose Pim, or how much this situation controls my life. But then we meet the above-mentioned Edwin, a fellow sufferer, and his wife Birgit. Edwin was several months ahead of Pim in the treatment.

> Birgit and I meet occasionally and app a lot. 'Does Edwin have a stem cell donor?' 'Pim's brother was also not a match...' 'How is it going with the second round of treatment?' 'Are the blood values rising yet?' 'When can he go home?' 'Edwin has blood poisoning.' 'Pim has an inexplicable fever'. 'Hey, I see that Pim is back in hospital!' 'When will you be there?' (Superbro, p. 74)

The contact with Birgit strengthened me in the communication with the medical professionals. And I remember very well Birgit visiting Pim, while Edwin was sleeping, spending a long time talking to him. These conversations with Birgit helped Pim more than all the information provided by the doctors.

Pim also found comfort in his bond with his friend Ronan, a young man suffering from another type of cancer and also treated at the LUMC hospital. Ronan unfortunately died by the time Pim was admitted for his stem cell transplant.

> Pim visited Ronan at home a few times during the summer. A bond formed between them: comrades, soldiers, fighting an invisible enemy in an unequal battle. Ronan was important to Pim. 'Only Ronan can know how I'm feeling', said Pim. (Superbro, p. 58)

5.3   Family and Friends

Of course, help also came from people around us: my colleagues and manager who allowed me to take time off to care for Pim, arranged a replacement for me and took over my projects. Help came from the university lecturer and the school mentor who showed sympathy with the situation facing Pim's brother and sister. The help came from family and friends: emotional, practical and even financial. We were and are truly grateful for all the help we received from these dear people.

However, their help mainly took place at home. We never considered the possibility asking for their help in the hospital, for example, in the conversations with the doctors. In hindsight that might have been a good idea, especially in times of real stress and fear. I suppose my father, if he had been in good shape, might have helped in the communication with the staff. But at the time of Pim's treatment, he was already too sick himself.

6   Lessons Learned

I like to think that I learned a lot about Pim's situation when he was hospitalized. I know better now what is required to communicate with medical staff and to participate in the hospital life, and maybe try to make a little difference in some situations. But I am not sure I would do it better now from how I did then. I can name list a few reasons for this belief.

First of all, in every life-threatening situation, it is very difficult to think clearly. Acting rationally is so hard when emotions take control. To my experience, noticing when your child is in danger blocks out most of rational thinking. Extreme stress and fear also diminish energy and power.

Secondly, as a patient and as the family of a patient, you are very dependent on the hospital staff and their manners. Being dependent makes you smile when you're angry, makes you silent when you should have spoken out loud, makes you follow the rules instead of jumping out of line. Diplomacy in general is of course the best way to act. But to be honest, filing complaints, breaking the rules or making a scene is much more effective. It felt to me that only in such conflict situations, did someone listen. As an adult, most of the times I tried the diplomatic way, but Pim couldn't care less. And as a result, he was seen as a burden.

Thirdly, as an individual it is extremely hard to stand up to bureaucracy. The hospital is so very big with so many rules and protocols, and there is such a strict hierarchy. Therefore it is almost useless to address individual staff members. These professionals have so few possibilities to change things themselves. Only the very brave and creative staff try to do so. I remember a nurse permitting one of Pim's friends to stay in the hospital overnight, which was not according to the rules, but exactly what Pim needed at that moment. I remember the physiotherapist allowing Pim to be in her gym, while she was practicing with other patients. Physical exercise was not included in Pim's treatment, but he really enjoyed being there, as he went to the gym at home all the time.

I know now what it takes to make a difference, no matter how small: being persistent, being assertive and most of all: being courageous. For future encounters with the hospital, I can only hope I have half the strength my son Pim has shown.

7   Reflection

My (Tineke Abma) reflection on Jet's narrative is grounded in the collaborative research project within the LUMC hospital. Jet was part of the collective and the group decided her story was a narrative each of them recognized. It was not an 'I-story' but a 'we-story.'

7.1   Slow Questions

One of the challenges in an academic hospital is that the participation of patients easily gets instrumentalized by technical and scientific frameworks in which control and mastery are paramount (Woelders 2019). Especially the attraction and heroism surrounding technology play an important role. Philosopher Kunneman (2017) talks about the 'seductive power' of modern technology: 'the phantasm to do away with all slow questions and exercising unlimited control over our lives and happiness'

(p. 188). 'Slow questions' are related to existential complexities when facing illness or death; slow questions cannot be fixed with technology. In a knowledge-intensive organization, these questions may shift into the background in the search for solutions and quick fixes by professionals.

The stories of Jet, Birgit and many others are full of 'slow questions'. This manifests itself in feelings of dependency and powerlessness. The story of Jet reveals that Pim's illness smashed away the solid ground for existence. This is primarily a physical condition associated with hunger, injury and disease, and with all associated emotions, such as pain, fear, sadness and despair. Jet talks about the 'losing control' and 'living in a daze.' Life seemed so malleable and plannable, but this is suddenly far away. What was self-evident is no longer so, no longer can Pim trust his own body. He and his family are face to face with an uncontrollable existential complexity and have absolutely no control over it. This is to be understood as a passive, 'suffering' relationship with the one's existence. The next quote captures it:

> Fighting is familiar, it is Pim's preferred strategy. During the first stage of the treatment Pim fought for all he was worth and only very occasionally displayed signs of choosing flight. Generally he bore the terrible chemotherapy like a soldier and after each session he pulled himself together and battled on. But now, after the stem cell transplant, Pim is frozen. It is pointless fighting what he is facing now. Flight is impossible. Freezing is all that is left: Pim is in survival mode. (Superbro, p. 68)

7.2   Quick Solutions Leave an Existential Residue

Faced with suffering professionals typically respond with technical solutions to fix the problem (Schön 1983). We can see this in the story of Jet; Pim is treated with stem cell transplantations and experimental treatments. He and his family are given the impression that the disease can be cured, and that the chances of recovery are relatively good given Pim's age. Everyone is, of course, happy to belief this. No one wants to give up; Pim is a fighter, and his family supports him in his fight.

Yet not everything can be tamed and solved. On the one hand, the confrontation with the vulnerability and dependence of the patient can strengthen the compassion among professionals and provide a fruitful soil for the effort to bring the patient safely back to normal life, away from the pain and the suffering, using all available technical means. On the other hand, these solutions can contribute to the suppression and denial of vulnerability, finiteness and loss of control. In other words, wanting to fix and solve the disease can also lead to reducing the moral and existential questions into technically solvable problems. Kunneman (2017) speaks in this regard of an 'existential residue' that is not amenable to objective and technical knowledge.

Many stories of patients, including Jet's narrative, are about the lack of attention and empathy for the patient and family, and for what cannot be solved, but needs to be worked through. The instrumental logic of the system focuses on efficiency and conflicts with the existential questions. Kunneman again:

An important characteristic of slow questions is the confrontation with the limits of fast, technical solutions and the necessity to 'muddle through,' to apply oneself to the 'labor of mourning,' to try and rewrite to a certain extent one's life history and envisage alternative ways to lead a meaningful life. (Kunneman 2017, p. 184)

As we can read in Jet's story patients and family are mostly on their own to grief and mourn about what is lost and cannot be repaired. The specialist nurse is an exception in Jet's story. He is taking enough time to listen and understand Pim as a person. Pim feels seen and heard by this nurse. This is also the case with some fellow sufferers and their family members who become friends, as well as with family and friends.

7.3   In-Between Space for Moral-Relational Learning

The encouraging message from our PAR project is that within the hospital context an in-between space can arise from building up a collective based on mutual relationships, respect and trust. Such a collective of patients, family, doctors, nurses and researchers can attend to and explore the slow questions with each other. Slow questions are then not pushed back to the lifeworld of patients and family, as in the case of Jet's story, but become connected with and embedded in the high technological context. This requires courage from patients, nurses, doctors and researchers to share their vulnerabilities, doubts and uncertainties, and to engage and facilitate these kinds of moral-relational learning processes to prevent participation from being reduced to a fixed format that describes who does what, in which roles are defined and in which tasks and responsibilities are laid down. Participation begins and ends with sharing experiences and exploring slow questions that have an existential and moral dimension.

The knowledge that arises in such a process of co-creation can be described as mode-3 knowledge. While mode-1 knowledge is the outcome of experts who strive for truth-finding through objective methods, and mode-2 knowledge is aimed at practical-instrumental application, mode-3 knowledge can be characterized as practical wisdom that arises in the context of knowledge-intensive organizations. In a postmodern society, organizations are characterized by creative frictions and a plurality of moral perspectives and existential scripts. Learning to act well in such a context requires and generates a different type of knowledge when a moral-relational learning process starts. As challenging as it may be, that is precisely where co-creation is so much needed:

In these domains, they [professionals] are also in need of inspiration and of moral and existential insights that can help them find more adequate ways of dealing with the complex mixtures of technical, strategic and moral questions confronting them. (Kunneman 2017, p. 195)

References

Abma TA, Banks S, Cook T, Dias S, Madsen W, Springett J, Wright M. Participatory research for health and social well-being. Cham: Springer; 2019.

Kunneman H. Amor complexitatis. Bouwstenen voor een kritisch humanisme. Deel 2. Amsterdam: Humanistic University Press; 2017.

Schön D. The reflective practitioner. Arena: Ashgate Publishing Limited; 1983.

Van der Voet J. Superbro, Den Haag. A printed English translation is for sale via www.bol.com; search for 'Superbro English version'. 2020.

Woelders S. Power-full patient participation. Opening spaces for silenced knowledge. Ridderkerk: Ridderprint BV; 2019.

Living with Anxiety and Severe Depression

Philip Leicester

Abstract This chapter describes my own experience growing up with anxiety, compulsory obsessive disorder, severe depression, and obsessive personality disorder. This has led me towards research aimed at helping those with low health literacy to self-manage their own conditions of anxiety and major depression through the development of an infographic.

Keywords Depression · Anxiety · Infographic · Low health literacy

1 Childhood

For as long as I can remember I have been sensitive, quiet, and anxious. Throughout my childhood I had a sense of fear which would come and go for no apparent reason. Physical and psychological abuse from my dad often simply because I was the eldest did little to allay the fear. For many years, my anxiety went undiagnosed, but to me and my parents, it was considered part of my behaviour and who I was. I was never examined as a child for anything which may have explained my nervous condition. One day, at 11 years of age, I suddenly felt a burning sensation in my stomach followed by complete stiffness of my body before blacking out. During this period, I felt I was spiralling clockwise through a vortex, clinging on tightly. When I emerged, I saw my chair had tipped sideways onto the floor. My mother and grandmother were trying desperately to pick me up.

The second epileptic episode happened 5 months later when my dad was cutting my hair. Just as I was beginning to fall, my dad grabbed me and carried me to my bed until the seizure had passed. My first experience with an electrocardiograph (EEG) was in 1971 at a large Melbourne Hospital. I sat in a large, padded chair with wires all around me that frightened mum. The neurologist diagnosed epileptic activity due to gaps within the communication region of my brain. I was told that I could

P. Leicester (✉)
Centre for Smart Analytics, Federation University Australia, Mt. Helen, VIC, Australia

A. Stranieri et al. (eds.), *Research Partners with Lived Experience*,
https://doi.org/10.1007/978-981-97-0033-2_13

do anything anyone else could, but it would take twice as long to complete! I was also prescribed anticonvulsive medication. My childhood recollection was that tests revealed I had a learning development delay and that some of my brain wave activity had similarities with juvenile delinquents. This was disturbing news at the time, but I can assure the reader that I have never committed any acts of juvenile delinquency!

I had little understanding of what was happening to me during my early years. The only resources available were family medical books and encyclopaedias. It wasn't until some years later that my understanding of epilepsy deepened through access to a broader range of relevant material. Amongst other things I learnt that epilepsy has a detrimental impact on social, vocational, and psychological functioning for numerous patients. I learnt that epilepsy was common especially in adolescence (Liu et al. 2022). Those with epilepsy tend to have lower educational achievements, lower annual salaries, and diminished health status compared with non-epileptic patients (Elliott et al. 2009).

2   Anxiety and Depression Breakdowns

I was 24 when I had my first nervous breakdown. A psychiatrist diagnosed acute anxiety and I was prescribed anti-anxiety drugs, beta-blockers, and anti-depressive medication. During this time, I felt completely lost, unable to concentrate, gripped with excessive worry about the future along with nightmares about dying on the operating table before turning thirty. I was also washing my hands repeatedly for no reason, always repeatedly checking what I had done before leaving the house, as well as repeatedly pacing due to my anxiety. It would take 5 years and a relocation with my family from a major city to a regional area before symptoms reduced. My psychiatrist recommended that I take up Eastern practices of yoga and meditation to manage acute anxiety. Pulling a rubber band around my wrist distracted my mind from bad thoughts.

One night a week, I was learning the techniques of Pranayama Hatha Yoga and Transcendental Meditation to look inward. I continued practicing these techniques each day until my mental health had resumed some balance and my fears had subsided substantially. Whenever I felt anxious or my thoughts were becoming irrational I would meditate.

In 2004, I had a second breakdown, more severe than the first and was referred to a new psychiatrist. His diagnosis was major depression, anxiety with obsessive compulsive personality disorder (OCDP). OCDP is a personality disorder that encompasses extreme neatness, order, and perfectionism. Those suffering from OCDP have no idea that there is anything wrong. This condition affects more men than women, especially those with existing mental health conditions (Mathis et al. 2011).

I became totally withdrawn and lost interest in activities that were once interesting. I was no longer taking part in family gatherings. I had become completely lost within myself with a sense of helplessness, uselessness, low self-esteem, low confidence, irregular thought patterns along with difficulty sleeping. Over the years, while my symptoms improved, I would continue to grapple with this. I spoke with my psychiatrist about studying to focus my mind and quell the ongoing brooding. Three years later as part of my "self-imposed education" therapy I commenced a master's coursework degree in information systems which I successfully completed in 2009. This enabled me to become a member of the university's chapter of the Golden Key honor society (https://www.goldenkey.org). This was a great accomplishment for me and boosted my confidence that I had the necessary academic qualities to pursue studies further towards research that might realise a benefit for others. I enrolled in a Graduate Diploma in Advanced Computing that was equivalent to an honours degree with a research component that could lead to a PhD. My research would revolve around health informatics. My personal experience with severe depression would become the topic of my research.

In 2011, I was admitted into a private hospital for the first time for a 2-week period to have a break away from home. It was during this time that I first learnt a great deal about my condition and the techniques of self-awareness, emotional intelligence, meditation (mindfulness), diet, medications, causes of depression and anxiety, as well as the physical symptoms produced by mental illnesses. The importance of the techniques had an immense effect on me and the self-management in dealing with my mental illness. This psychological tool kit would assist me in managing my own mental health and would provide me with the necessary information to assist others with the same mental conditions in some form in the future. Over the next 9 years I would encounter six more admissions for changes in medication and a relapse of my illness to severe depression.

3 Research

At the age of 54, I was granted a scholarship in a West Australian university to work on a topic chosen for me that involved designing a mobile application. I was very anxious. My father was angry with me for going to Perth. Within the year, I withdrew and returned home. The following year I enrolled in a PhD programme at a regional university, the University of Ballarat (now Federation University). I wanted to work on a topic that might help those who had problems with mental illness. It was suggested to me by my supervisor Associate Professor Andrew Straneri that I focus my research on the effects low health literacy had on individuals dealing with depression and anxiety issues since I had lived, personal experience since childhood. At the University of Ballarat, I was lucky enough to have a team of academics to support me. My experience with mental illness led me to investigate the effects that low health literacy had on individuals/patients suffering from mental illness and how the use of infographics could assist these individuals/patients with the self-management of their condition.

There are many barriers that adults with low health literacy (LHL) encounter that restricts them from managing their chronic condition. Barriers include low education standards, low socio-economic background, language and cultural differences, cognitive impairment, mental illness, and computer illiteracy (Kountz 2009; Torpy et al. 2011). Those with LHL have difficulty with medical jargon, understanding health information such as written medical instructions and completing health insurance forms. They are prone to greater risks of hospitalization with longer periods of admittance and frequently have more visits to emergency departments due to their poorer health status (Kountz 2009; Torpy et al. 2011). Although there has been much research undertaken on the link between health literacy and patient empowerment, there has been little research in establishing methods that will enable those with low health literacy (LHL) to manage their conditions.

According to studies (McCaffery et al. 2013), combining pictorial and written material on health information can be helpful in terms of patient cognitive processes of comprehension, retention, and adherence on patients with low health literacy (LHL) skills (Peregrin 2010). The type of visual infographics for LHL patients must be simple (easy to comprehend and understand) to cater for ease of understanding.

4 Infographics

The application of infographics is especially important in the communication of health information to those with LHL as the quality of the infographic will have a direct impact on their understanding of the visual information being communicated. For LHL patients to self-manage their depression, they first need to understand the condition, be aware of the symptoms, follow medication instructions, undertake some form of activity, and maintain regular visits to their therapist. The infographic that I initially designed consisted of a circle with categories each with a specific role and links to other pages containing infographic information and videos that would help them understand more about their anxiety and depression. Each category had a specific colour scheme representing the type of information being provided. The infographic was designed to contain the various areas important for self-management for severe depression and anxiety which I adopted in dealing with my own mental health illnesses.

5 Epilogue

During my time as a research student, I had to overcome many obstacles with my physical and mental health which forced me to have a great deal of time away from studies making it difficult to pick up from I left off from each break. Since the start of my research in 2014, I endured two knee replacements, a right shoulder repair, numerous arthroscopes, and a few stays at a hospital for my mental health. In 2019,

Mum was in the last stage of a terminal illness and maintaining research and my mental balance became impossible. After withdrawing from university, my mental health declined quickly and I was re-admitted to hospital in 2020 following suicidal thoughts. During the 4 weeks I was admitted, I took to song writing which enabled me to express my emotions and my creative side. Over a period of 12 months, I wrote the lyrics to 30 songs. The first song I wrote is titled The Lonely Trail.

This Lonely Trail

At the age of seven this trail began (C to EM)
Born from anxiety and fear
A lonely boy where isolation became the norm
From the protective wall that he would endear

Chorus

This lonely trail (AM)
He would follow (EM)
Where strangers would pass him by (G to D)
A trail thrusted upon him (AM to EM)
For his entire life (G to AM)
[Through his teenage years]
[He was bullied at school]
At Home where strict discipline was abound
Would escalate his nervousness
Not knowing why such cruelty and pain
Withdrew him further into his imagination

Chorus

This lonely trail
He would follow
Where strangers would pass him by
A trail thrusted upon him
For his entire life
[As the years went by]
[He saw the natural coldness of life]
[Where people are prisoners]
[Separated from their precious things]
He continues on this solidarity path
To where no one knows
Thou pleasant and friendly along his journey (D to AM)
He is different from those around him (AM)
Just keeps on walking this lonely trail (G to D)

Chorus

[This lonely trail] (AM)
[He would follow] (EM)
[Where strangers would pass him] by (G to D)
[As if there were no tomorrow] (AM to EM)
[In the sunshine of his life] (G to D)
[This lonely trail]
[He would follow]
[Where strangers would pass him by]
[A trail thrusted upon him]
[For his entire life]

In 2020, I was admitted for 2 weeks to undergo 28 sessions of cranial magnetic therapy which unfortunately didn't work. I also underwent some neurological testing as I had experienced some sleep paralysis and hallucinations at home and was concerned that there might be some abnormal physical brain activity. The neurological tests cleared me of any neurological physical disturbances but did show that my amygdala was elongated with some mild tremors in both hands.

Mum passed away at home in 2020 and I was re-admitted into hospital in October to deal with grief. It was in May of that year that I wrote a song dedicated to her. The song was titled Mother's Love.

Mother's Love

[Verse 1]
On Mother's Day we celebrate the sacrifices
That mother's make every day
Her maternal instincts
That she reacts upon each day
She is our teacher, our protector, our nursemaid
And our spiritual guide
[Chorus]
A mother's love knows no bounds
For her love is simply divine
A love that has no conditions
For this love is her life
That is a mother's love

[Verse 2]
She feeds us, clothes us
And changes with us
As we walk the road of life
She inspires us and is proud of us
In what we do
Her wisdom and dedication is her soul
[Chorus]
A mother's love knows no bounds
For her love is simply divine
A love that has no conditions
For this love is her life
That is a mother's love

[Verse 3]
As the years go by while she ages
In the autumn of her life
The coldness of winter finally takes her
Causing part of us to die
For the memories will stay with us
For a mother's love never dies
[Chorus]
A mother's love knows no bounds
For her love is simply divine
A love that has no conditions
For this love is her life
That is a mother's love

[Chorus]
A mother's love knows no bounds
For her love is simply divine
A love that has no conditions
For this love is her life
That is a mother's love

Nine months later, in 2021, my dad passed away from a stroke. I again had a 2-week stay in hospital to deal with my grief. By this time, I had completely stopped song writing and any other forms of creativity as I was adjusting to life without them.

Unfortunately, I didn't complete my research into the impact of infographics on those with low health literacy. I'm confident that infographics can help those with low health literacy deal the symptoms and causes of their anxiety and depression.

Since moving to a small rural town in 2022, I find myself totally changed within, where my thoughts and memory have completely altered. Most of the time I'm just sitting in my recliner watching TV and falling asleep in the afternoon. I no longer do meditation or any other self-helping activity since I no longer have the inclination and interest. This bothers me very much as I know what I should be doing, but I don't know why this has happened. The biggest problem is boredom, depressive laziness, and a lack of determination to do anything about it. I know extremely well that only I can improve my situation otherwise, in the end, my life will be cut short.

I trust that this chapter of my experience in dealing with severe depression and anxiety will provide some benefit to readers. I also hope that this article will provide some understanding on how mental illness affects and helps to eradicate the stigma still associated with it. Society needs to know that there is nothing to fear from mental illness, that it is an illness and nothing more.

I thank very much Associate Professor Andrew Stranieri and Dr. Sally Firmin for asking me to participate in the writing of this book. I was incredibly grateful to be of assistance.

References

Elliott JO, Lu B, Shneker BF, Moore JL, McAuley JW. The impact of 'social determinants of health'on epilepsy prevalence and reported medication use. Epilepsy Res. 2009;84(2-3):135–45.

Kountz DS. Strategies for improving low health literacy. Postgrad Med. 2009;121(5):171–7.

Liu X, Sun X, Sun C, Zou M, Chen Y, Huang J, Chen W-X. Prevalence of epilepsy in autism spectrum disorders: a systematic review and meta-analysis. Autism. 2022;26(1):33–50.

Mathis MAD, Alvarenga PD, Funaro G, Torresan RC, Moraes I, Torres AR, Hounie AG. Gender differences in obsessive-compulsive disorder: a literature review. Braz J Psychiatry. 2011;33:390–9.

McCaffery KJ, Holmes-Rovner M, Smith SK, Rovner D, Nutbeam D, Clayman ML, Sheridan SL. Addressing health literacy in patient decision aids. BMC Med Inform Decis Mak. 2013;13(2):1–14.

Peregrin T. Picture this: visual cues enhance health education messages for people with low literacy skills. J Am Diet Assoc. 2010;110(5):28–32.

Torpy JM, Burke AE, Golub RM. Health literacy. JAMA. 2011;306(10):1158.

It's in Your Head!

Armita Zarnegar

Abstract This story covers a period of my life between 2014 and 2017. It is the story of a 41-year-old middle eastern woman who experienced prejudice combined with a limited way of thinking in the medical system. I was injured during an aged-care shift while assisting a paraplegic patient move from his bed to a wheelchair. For 18 months following my injury, I suffered from chronic pain with no diagnosis. During this time, I made several attempts to gain a diagnosis and proper treatment. The account of my last unsuccessful attempt is described here as well as the journey toward a satisfactory outcome. After 18 months of visiting specialists and trying several treatment options, I decided to take the matter into my own hands and engaged in research to establish a way out of my disabling, chronic pain. My journey has had a successful outcome as I managed to find a diagnosis and a treatment plan. Currently, I am living a relatively normal life. This experience has empowered and inspired me to use my skills as a computer science researcher in the health and medicine domain and enabled me to commence a pathway to Health Informatics research.

Keywords Patient experience · Patient journey · Thoracic nerve injury · Chronic pain · Lived experience · Psychosomatic pain

1 Diagnosis: "Psychosomatic Pain"

I was looking at his face, but the doctor was not paying attention to me, nor the pile of imaging and medical documents I had placed on my lap. Instead, he was doing something on his computer. He finally finished and turned back to me to ask why I had come to him and what was wrong. I started to explain how the pain in my right armpit spread up my back to my shoulder, how I had lost strength in my entire arm,

A. Zarnegar (✉)
School of Science, Computing and Engineering Technologies, Swinburne University of Technology, Melbourne, VIC, Australia
e-mail: azarnegar@swin.edu.au

© The Author(s), under exclusive license to Springer Nature Singapore Pte Ltd. 2024
A. Stranieri et al. (eds.), *Research Partners with Lived Experience*,
https://doi.org/10.1007/978-981-97-0033-2_14

and how it all started when helping transfer a paraplegic patient from his bed to a wheelchair.

He asked me where I came from, and I told him it was Iran. He said, "Ok, so you must have experienced war there? Is that the reason you moved here?" I told him that was not the reason and that when I moved to Australia, there was no war in Iran, but there had been a war between Iran and Iraq when I was a child. "So, you experienced war as a child!" he exclaimed. I nodded in agreeance, although it was not strictly true.

The doctor kept asking me if it was hard to live in Australia as an immigrant and I started wondering where these questions were leading. This seemed beyond simple curiosity or small talk between a doctor and a patient. I agreed that immigration is hard, but then I continued by asking, "Would you like to look at all my medical imaging?" He said, "no, just stand up and try to raise your hand straight up." I did what he asked, and then he requested another two movements which I performed.

Finally, he stopped and said, "Ok, that is all." I was puzzled and asked him what his diagnosis was. He answered, "have you heard about psychosomatic pain? You had been traumatized in Iran because of the war so one day your brain decided to feel the pain, many years later." I was shocked by what he claimed to be the cause of my pain. I looked at him and said, "I am telling you, I lifted a patient, and while doing that, I felt something "pop" in my armpit and this is not something that I made up!". He then said, "but that was a minor injury, and you should be healed by now. Perhaps the pain of that injury triggered your traumatized brain to feel the pain." I asked how he could know this without even checking the results of my diagnostic tests and imaging. At this point, he stood up and told me there was nothing he could do for me, and I needed to see a psychiatrist. He then walked to the door, opened it and asked me to leave.

I walked out of his office, shaking. At the front desk, the receptionist asked me to pay the doctor's consultation fee of $320 (40% of my weekly average salary). I was almost in tears, but I took out my credit card and paid the money, then walked away slowly.

In the car I felt tears rolling down my cheeks. I rested my head on the steering wheel and cried aloud, a long cry. I cried for my entire life, for the fact that I would be judged and labeled for the rest of my life in Australia simply because I came from the Middle East; I cried for my loneliness as a single mum in a foreign country without family or friends; for experiencing such prejudices that hindered me from receiving proper and impartial medical treatment; for the bullying and discrimination that I had experienced at work, which resulted in this disabling injury; and lastly I cried for my 7-year-old daughter who had to rely on a mum with a disability struggling to manage all their day to day needs. Incidentally, I found out on the day of the incident that the hoist used by the patient was broken and they lied to me telling me that the patient had been assessed as being able to be transferred without a hoist.

Suddenly, in thinking about my daughter, I realized I was running late to pick her up. I could not afford the time to cry or indulge in self-pity, I had a child dependent on me for everything. In a panic, I rushed to her school to pick her up.

At school, I hid in a corner as my face was puffy and red. My daughter noticed the redness in my nose and eyes and asked me if I was all right. I reassured her, "yes, it is not important. I just had a bad day, and my arm hurts, as usual." I saw sadness in her pretty, big, brown eyes, but she did not say anything. It seems that she was used to feeling sad because of me. Since my injury, I have been crying on and off, sometimes she would cry with me trying to console me by telling me not to worry as she would help take care of me.

That night after making dinner, clearing up and putting my daughter to bed, I sat down and looked at my photo album, the only memento I had brought with me from all those years of living in Iran. I felt nostalgic and wished to be there with people like myself. People who do not know much about "psychosomatic pain" or the term "traumatized" but have been experiencing war and conflict for many years. The friendly, hospitable, and smart people of my homeland. I took my phone and tried to ring my dad. There was no answer. Tears streamed down my cheeks; I closed my eyes and fell asleep.

That night was a turning point and the start of a journey having decided to seek a medical opinion elsewhere. The specialist previously mentioned was the seventh I had seen in the 18 months after the incident in 2014 that left me with chronic pain.

The background to all this was that in 2014 I was working for a research center providing IT services. My contract was coming to an end. Finding a job with a bio-informatics PhD would take some time, so I thought of getting a certificate in Aged Care as I have always enjoyed dealing with older adults. This would enable me to secure an income when needed. As I had a full-time job, I had to find a place to study after work and on weekends. I found a company that let me work for them with training sessions in the evening and shifts to work during the weekends. Unfortunately, the manager was quite a bully, and the training provided lacked any practical component.

One day, early in the morning I was sent to a shift, not realising what was ahead for me. I did not know that I was being sent to provide care for a disabled patient who happened to be a paraplegic. My previous clients were all elderly people as my training was in aged-care. I rang the company to ask what to do with him as I had no training and experience dealing with this disability and the company told me that I would be fine if I just followed the patient's instructions.

The patient asked me to help him manually transfer from the bed to the wheel-chair. I asked him whether he had a hoist (not that I knew how to operate one). He replied no and said that he only needed some assistance sometimes. I accepted this and attempted to transfer him. It was then when he almost collapsed on me, and me trying to hold him that I felt the "pop" in my armpit. Once the shift was almost over and the patient was about to go to work, he told me to open a door and remove the hoist and leave it outside as people were coming to take it for repair!

I reported the incident and the nature of pain to the manager on the same day, only to face her anger, having her blame me for everything. I did not take my injury seriously until the pain was unbearable, even with painkillers, so I went to see a GP. My first GP kept telling me that there was no muscle where I was pointing, and

I should gradually get better. He referred me to a physiotherapist. In total I saw my GP three times regarding this pain.

I had a couple of physiotherapy sessions before changing to another GP. By the time I changed my GP which was about 2 months after the incident, I received a referral to see a neurologist specialist who gave me an appointment in about 6 weeks. Following this appointment, I then waited more than 3 weeks for an MRI. By this time it was already three and a half months since the incident and my arm was still in constant pain.

Given the findings of the MRI (some torn muscles) the neurologist then decided that I was best to be under the care of an Orthopedic surgeon. I saw a number of Orthopedic surgeons followed by two sports medicine physicians. The sixth specialist told me that my first MRI was conducted too late, making any diagnosis difficult. During the 15 months following the incident, I had many physiotherapy sessions (targeted at my shoulder) along with hydrotherapy, chiropractic and acupuncture treatments, but there was no improvement.

I had to stop all of these sessions due to the pain in my arm. I could not even keep my arms over the desk for more than an hour to type or do computer work. After that hour, I was in pain for a couple more hours and any subsequent attempt to sit at a desk was even shorter than an hour. To help with this, I requested a standing desk only to be sent for a medical assessment which identified me as not fit for work. This request subsequently led to my dismissal.

During the first 18 months after my injury, when I suffered from chronic pain, was unemployed, and struggled to hold a nozzle to fill up my car or carry my shopping bags I tried several painkillers none of which worked and one led to a strong allergic reaction and kidney pain for weeks. I started searching for ways to deal with pain online and what I found, apart from a bunch of illegal drugs, were postings from those with chronic pain, full of suicidal thoughts and suggestions of ways to end your life. Honestly, it crossed my mind that I could not live with this pain forever but the fact that I had my daughter whose life depended on me made me push those thoughts away. The prospect of living with chronic pain was like living in hell with no end; at some point, one starts thinking about ways to end it.

In an attempt to find a way out of this situation I started on my journey into research. Based on reading scientific literature, I discovered that MRI diagnostic accuracy for the thoracic area (the location of my pain) is only around 60%. Interestingly, the specialists who I visited did not know about this and kept telling me that MRI is pretty accurate. I also investigated different MRI techniques to find if there is any way to identify my problem using different MRI parameters or protocols. I read many papers in this area and compared their findings which progressed to my interest and research in systematic review (Khalil et al. 2022). At the same time, I started web searching or "googling" hospitals and clinics worldwide to find medical opinions outside of Australia. I investigated clinics in Germany (Health Service Germany 2015) and the Mayo Clinic (Mayo Clinic 2015) in New York, authoring a few emails to explore treatment options available at these facilities. Ultimately, I organized a visit to a hospital in Germany and arranged a stopover in Iran to visit my dad, who had not been well.

2   A Lonely Journey

In October 2015, I flew to Iran. My dad's condition was worse than I was expecting. As a stereotypical man, he refused to go to a doctor and I had to push him and book appointments. My dad was diagnosed with stage 4 intestinal cancer two weeks after my arrival. He had required emergency surgery as a tumor was blocking his intestine. A quick change of plan was needed, so I decided to stay in Iran while my dad underwent surgery and chemotherapy. During that time, I took the opportunity to consult Orthopedic surgeons and other specialists for my own condition. I had no success with the first one, but the second specialist, who was an out of-the-box thinker (Bahman Hospital 2015), asked if a nerve conduction study had been performed in my upper back area. I replied that I had.

He said that the nerve test in that area is tricky and maybe it would be worth repeating. He referred me to a neurologist for a thorough assessment and diagnosis. The neurologist was thorough, telling me he sources his needles from Switzerland as they are thinner and more accurate. He managed to detect weakness in the thoracic nerve in my upper back and this was the first time that anybody had suggested a diagnosis for my problem. I went back to the Orthopedic surgeon with this new found diagnosis. He started by saying, "There is no surgical solution for your problem; my only recommendation is targeted and intense physiotherapy." I replied to him, "but I did tons of physio sessions, and they did not change anything for me." He said, "this time it is going to be different; just trust me; you now have a diagnosis, go there and follow their advice."

The physio clinic in Iran was something unexpected. I had not seen anything like this in Australia. The principal physiotherapist had a long consultation with me and gave me a targeted program together with a tour of his facility "You will start with ultrasound each day, then an hour and a half of exercises, followed by cold laser," He also said, "I might apply dry needling at the beginning for the first few sessions. It will all take 3 hours, and you will need to attend here three times a week." I asked, "How long do I need to do this?" He replied, "It takes at least a couple of months until you start seeing results."

I should confess that I was very skeptical when I started that program. However, it took me less than a month to notice the difference. Finally, something worked! Meanwhile, I was attending these physio sessions, and many things were happening at a personal level and two months after I started the physio, I had to leave Iran suddenly and return to Australia. Regrettably, a nasty divorce then ensued.

Thankfully, though my chronic pain had disappeared, I stopped taking pain medications and my quality of life had improved. After returning, I tried to continue with some exercises at home, but soon, due to ongoing stressors I stopped following the routine. I was expecting that things would become worse again, but fortunately, they did not. The effect of those physio sessions back in Iran have lasted well. A couple of weeks after I had arrived back in Australia, I started a pain management program that my GP had referred me to before I left for Iran. I decided to attend the program in the event that the pain returned. Incidentally, I still felt pain when lifting heavy objects, changing sheets or vacuuming. The pain program was not entirely a waste of time; at least, as it taught me to pace myself. The psychologist and physio were limited to a couple of sessions and were not remarkably effective from my point of view.

My dad passed away more than a year after his diagnosis. A few months after his passing, I started working as a casual academic on a part-time basis. I increased my workload over the following 3 years and then started working full-time. Now, I am living almost a normal life. I cannot do some things around the house without feeling pain, such as vacuum cleaning, changing sheets or lifting heavy items but apart from that, I am managing most of the tasks in my everyday life thanks to God and my perseverance to find an answer. I am aware that my shoulders are degrading in functionality as a side effect of my primary injury, and my body has lost its symmetry. I have accepted that. I am counting my blessings and am thankful to God for my current life.

There is another part of this story that is worth mentioning and it involves a protracted legal battle involving a worker's compensation battle with an insurance company. Early on, lawyers advised me to give up on a bullying claim against my employer and persevere with the worker's compensation claim as the process of proving an employer's fault it is often too difficult. All the details in this legal battle would require a lengthy explanation and outside the intention of the article. In summary though, I hardly received a quarter of the cost of my medical expenses and some of my wages before I gave up. For those unfamiliar with the world of worker's compensation it is a messy area of the law and as my lawyer once said, "It is not about justice or fairness but what you can achieve considering the law." Many workers suffer awfully by corrupt insurance companies who reject more than 80% of claims (Worksafe Queensland 2021). I really hope someone does something about this as I have seen many injured workers suffer to the point of becoming suicidal due to the treatment they receive in the system. In all, my case took more 5 years to be resolved and a considerable amount of mental distress.

3   Conclusion

I used to work in the IT industry before my injury, however, my injury made it impossible for me to maintain a full-time job. Having a PhD qualification already, I started working as a casual academic. I enjoyed teaching, but I was inspired to use IT and technology to empower people to seek information for themselves and not blindly accept doctors' opinions. Coming from an academic background, I found the approach of some doctors to patient treatment not to be scientific. It seems some doctors believe: "our tests show nothing is wrong with you, so you should be fine." For me it appears that when a test does not show anything, but evidence and symptoms are present, it implies that the tests cannot capture reality. Thus, it is Ok to say I do not know rather than say "you should be fine" or even worse "it is all in your head, it is psychosomatic pain!".

I am sure my experience is not an isolated one in the western medical system. Patients approach clinicians to find answers to their pain and problems but in some cases, like mine, they face judgment and prejudice that only exacerbate their pain and suffering. The assumption by some medical professionals is that they know it all and there is a limited mindset of discovery or second-guessing of the assumptions. Based on my experience, some are not up to date with the latest medical research and seem to produce an answer based on the firm belief that this system never fails and has answers for everything. Patients with complex cases/conditions suffer in this model, feeling hopeless and are not believed. Their feelings, thoughts, and experiences are commonly ignored. It is as though all that is needed to know about a patient's body is recorded in medical texts or the minds of doctors and the patient's experience is ignored or considered misleading.

On the personal level, after the dust settled, I was keen to use my knowledge of technology and informatics in the health domain. My PhD was in the Bioinformatics domain and I published a few papers in that area (Zarnegar et al. 2009, 2016) but after my injury and reading a lot of medical papers, I decided to shift to the Health Informatics area and published a few of papers in that domain (Stranieri et al. 2022; Zarnegar 2023). Specifically, I was interested in Systematic reviews and automation tools to make these reviews faster. During those years of dealing with my medical issue, I read many papers, and this made me interested in tools to automate the literature review process which involved developing Natural Language Processing (NLP) and machine learning tools (Ofoghi and Zarnegar 2021). Currently I am a lecturer in Computer Science and my research interests are systematic review and digital health.

Acknowledgment I would like to thank Dr. Shahrokh Moradi for changing my life, for believing and listening to his patients and thinking out of the box to find a diagnosis for me. I would also like to thank Dr. Dayani the physiotherapist who helped me with his plan to transform my body and enable me to get rid of the disabling chronic pain that I had previously. Finally, Associate Professor Andrew Stranieri, a mentor, friend and a great researcher for his ongoing support and advice on this journey.

References

Bahman Hospital. Dr Sharokh Moradi. 2015. Retrieved from Bahman: http://bahmanhospital.ir/english/index.php/doctors.html.

Health Service Germany. 2015. Retrieved from Surgical Experts: www.surgical-experts.de.

Khalil H, Ameen D, Zarnegar A. Tools to support the automation of systematic reviews: a scoping review. J Clin Epidemiol. 2022;144:22–42.

Mayo Clinic. Mayo clinic. 2015. Retrieved from Mayo Clinic: https://www.mayoclinic.org/.

Ofoghi B, Zarnegar A. Answer passage ranking enhancement using shallow linguistic features. In: Modeling decisions for artificial intelligence: 18th international conference. Umeå: Springer; 2021. p. 27–30.

Stranieri A, Venkatraman S, Minicz J, Zarnegar A, Firmin S, Jelinek H. Emerging point of care devices and artificial intelligence: prospects and challenges for public health. Smart Health. 2022;2022:100279.

WorkSafe Queensland. 2021. https://www.worksafe.qld.gov.au/__data/assets/pdf_file/0025/89602/
   workers-compensation-scheme-statistics-202021-full-report.pdf.

Zarnegar A. Point-of-care devices in healthcare: a public health perspective. In: Current and future
   trends in health and medical informatics. Cham: Springer; 2023.

Zarnegar A, Vamplew P, Stranieri A. Inference of gene expression networks using memetic gene
   expression programming. In: Proceedings of the Thirty-Second Australasian Conference on
   Computer Science, vol. 91. Sydney: Australian Computer Society; 2009. p. 29–36.

Zarnegar A, Vamplew P, Stranieri A, Jelinek H. A heuristic gene regulatory networks model for
   cardiac function and pathology. In: 2016 computing in cardiology conference (CinC). IEEE:
   Piscataway; 2016. p. 353–5.

How Lived Experience Mediated My Gold, Ribbons, Puzzles and Morals Research Motivations: A Reflective Introspection

Andrew Stranieri

Abstract Studies on factors that motivate researchers conclude that financial rewards, recognition, curiosity and a desire to contribute; the so-called, *Gold, Ribbons, Puzzle* and *Morals* motivating factors, combine to explain why individuals start and continue to be researchers. Lived experience with significant, often life-changing events as a patient, carer, victim, or bystander has motivated many, directly or indirectly, including me, to become researchers. In this chapter, I draw on introspection to examine my journey through 25 years of research experience in university settings. I use concepts from dual systems theories that identify intuition and cognition as two processes that come together to explain how key events and situations in life have influenced my decisions. This illustrates how critical events have mediated the *Gold*, *Ribbon*, *Puzzle* and *Morals* factors that were motivating my research efforts.

1 Introduction

Collaborations between patients with personal, intense experience with a condition and researchers investigating the condition have increased in recent years (Kirwan et al. 2017). Other intense experiences, such as those associated with, violence, bullying or racism can also be strong motivating factors toward the conduct of research. Research collaborations in the medical domain can take many forms: patients can engage with researchers by participating in literature reviews, helping to design studies, interpretating results, and writing articles (Abma 2019). Patients also commence research degrees, participate in studies as co-investigators, or initiate new studies and join research networks. Patients have also participated by helping to analyse data (Clarke et al. 2018).

A. Stranieri (✉)
Institute of Innovation, Science and Sustainability, Federation University, Ballarat, VIC, Australia
e-mail: a.stranieri@federation.edu.au

© The Author(s), under exclusive license to Springer Nature Singapore Pte Ltd. 2024
A. Stranieri et al. (eds.), *Research Partners with Lived Experience*,
https://doi.org/10.1007/978-981-97-0033-2_15

Patients as researchers enhance their empowerment and provide other researchers with a greater understanding of the condition under investigation (Abma 2019). However, many challenges have been identified when patients attempt to transition to becoming researchers: they are often not accepted as genuine researchers, sometimes mistrusted and need to demonstrate that their intense experiences will not impede their objectivity or introduce an unproductive sentimentality to explorations (Riggare 2020).

Lam (2015) examined scientists motivations to conduct research and identified a complex set of interacting factors categorised as reputational or career rewards, *Ribbon* factors, financial rewards, *Gold* factors and intrinsic curiosity and love of problem solving, labelled *Puzzle* factors. Van De Burgwal et al. (2019) found that many scientists in The Netherlands were additionally motivated by a sense of duty to grander causes including contributing to society and advancing knowledge. These motivators differed from *Gold, Ribbon* and *Puzzle* factors and were labelled *Moral* factors. Atta-Owusu and Fitjar (2022) demonstrated that contributing to the betterment of society explained researcher engagement to a greater extent than other factors though *Puzzle* factors were particularly strong motivators amongst entrepreneurial scientists who focus on commercially driven research (Suominen et al. 2021).

Gold and *Ribbon* factors are endorsed in modern university settings with publication and citation counts used as individual performance indicators, often linked directly to promotion opportunities. This has been criticised by Smyth et al. (2017) as creating excessively competitive and toxic academic environments. Joynson and Leyser (2015) also suggest that many institutional aspects of research in modern settings including excessive competition and focus on performance metrics discourages collaboration and creativity and thwarts the contribution to society motivation.

Intense lived experiences, such as those associated with medical conditions, violence, bullying or racism can also be a strong motivating factor toward the conduct of research. However, how the lived experience relates to other motivating factors is not well understood. The perspective advanced in this chapter juxtaposes the *Gold*, *Puzzle*, *Ribbon* and *Morals* factors against behaviour change theories presuming that the transition from non-researcher to researcher can be regarded as a significant behavioural change.

Pinder et al. (2018) points out that a multitude of approaches that explain behaviour and its change emphasise cognitive linkages between intentions, motivations and actions. Classical behaviour change theories surveyed by Kwasnicka et al. (2016) provide a chain starting from an intention to change behaviour, through triggering factors that stimulate intentions toward actions and sustain the behaviour change. However, Pinder et al. (2018) suggests that the landscape is more complex and, in practice includes idiosyncratic, situational and contextual factors that can be understood in terms of dual process theories.

Dual process theories advanced by Evans and Stanovich (2013), Kahneman (2011), and Strack and Deutsch (2004) contend that psychological processes derive from the interplay between two distinct processes, an intuitive, impulsive, limbic system processes and a rational, cognitive, higher cortex process. Processing brain waves during a judge's sentencing reasoning, Buckholtz et al. (2008) found that brain activation was initially observed in parts of the brain associated with intuitive processes then spreads to higher cortex regions more associated with thinking and then iterated between the two. Many studies in other contexts surveyed by Bellini-Leite (2022) have found evidence for dual process theory models and conclude an often overlooked theme; that decision making is embodied in specific contexts. Embodied cognition involves recognising that reasoning toward a decision involves a reasoner situated in a context at a point in time, drawing on intuition and rationality to arrive at a preferred decision.

An exercise in introspection of my own journey into computational intelligence research related to legal reasoning in the 1990's and transitioning into health informatics research in the 2000's interwoven with intense life events at critical points in time, leads me to suggest that a kind of embodied cognition led me to make decisions about my research efforts that felt right at the time, even though I may well have reached different decisions even weeks later. Historically regarded as methodologically flawed, introspection draws renewed attention (Burkart 2018). It is considered appropriate here as exploring researcher motivations is likely to be quite personal and nuanced. This reflection may reveal how intense experiences relate to the other motivating factors.

2   My Journey

There was little to suggest a research career lay ahead during my childhood years as a child of Italian immigrants to Australia, attending a non-academic, vocationally oriented secondary school. A lack of manual aptitude for any apprenticeship led me to meander into a university degree. Universities in Australia up to the late 1960s were relatively elite. Small numbers of students had the means to cover quite high fees and even fewer low-income students entered on academically based, fee waiver scholarships. In the 1970s a reformist government removed fees and opened tertiary education opportunities to many students like me, who had neither the funds nor the academic record.

Since the 1500s, a doctorate qualification has been required to teach law, medicine and philosophy at university (Moore 2018). In Australian universities in the 1970s, staff who had made an original contribution to knowledge recognised by the award of Doctor of Philosophy continued the tradition and combined research with teaching (Baptista et al. 2015). I can now imagine the transition that generation of staff had to make in order to accommodate the new cohorts of ragamuffin, non-traditional, low-income students.

I stumbled into a first-year science programme and was compelled, by my relatively poor vocational school grades to take subjects with low academic entry requirements. Ironically, psychology, was one of them. I immediately discovered a fascination with psychology inspired by a particularly passionate and accomplished professorial researcher who set the first-year students a challenging open-ended, self-directed, research-based assignment. My first foray into research was thoroughly exciting though I lacked the English expression, critical thinking and reading skills for my grades to reflect my endeavours. My interest in psychology spurred me to take an audacious step to transfer to a prestigious university's quite famous psychology degree. A senior tutor there, who had just been given notice, for his public excesses at late night rock venues that dominated the music scene in the 1980s, took delight in exercising discretion in admitting this vocational, migrant student with no grades to speak of, into the elite honours programme in second year, amidst a cohort of exceptionally academic students. Gleefully oblivious to the challenge or his motives, I enrolled in the Bachelor of Arts (Honours) degree. That quite extraordinary happenstance influenced many decades of my life.

In the honours programme that commenced in my second undergraduate year, I certainly struggled. One tutor, incredulous that I was a second-year Arts student who had never before written an essay, took the time to teach me how to write academically. The reading load was intense. Gradually, I came to know my fellow students, not as products of elite private schools but as people, and many as friends. After surviving for a year, I thought that I too, might make it through the third year and into the fourth, research-only year, even though I had come from a migrant and vocational background. I scraped into the fourth year, on appeal, however, a few days into the fourth-year research project, perhaps seeing I was going to be too much work, my supervisor dropped me. Senior staff tried to persuade me that this was not the dominant culture telling a migrant child he did not belong, but merely a set-back that allowed me to take a break and resume studies the following year with a new supervisor. However, rational and sage, this option ignored the anger, despondency and frustration that had overwhelmed me. I took great satisfaction in withdrawing from the degree, vowing to forever avoid circles I did not belong in.

For the next 5 years I travelled and worked many blue-collar jobs before re-training in the newly emerging profession of computing at a different, less elite university. Although I found little in computing that was particularly interesting, artificial intelligence and its application to legal reasoning was fascinating. My aptitude and enthusiasm led to an honours degree in computer science, as a mature age student, where I worked closely with lawyers to model their reasoning. This led to a scholarship to continue the work. By then, I had finally left the stream of blue-collar positions and had secured a mid-level paid public service administrative position. I had also partnered and my wife and I wanted to start a family so dropping the secure salary for a minimal PhD scholarship was irresponsible. However, seeing my excitement during the honours research and my lack of excitement going to work, my wife encouraged me to take up the scholarship. Though this felt irrational and irresponsible, intuitively it felt right. We dropped income substantially and I commenced doctoral research.

Soon after commencement, our newborn died from a rare congenital condition. Our public health physician dismissed my wife's intuitive concerns that something was wrong. A Chinese medicine practitioner directing Chi through my wife's body during pregnancy told her that events would unfold however they unfolded "worry or no worry—same".

After our baby's death, I found that I could not continue with something as trite as doctoral research. This was new proof that I did not belong in academia. I was unaware of the growing research in imposter syndrome that may have influenced my cognition at the time (Parkman 2016). Eventually, my feelings that I had dared to play outside my league and been punished for it gave way to a determination to complete the research as best I could as a dedication to our first child. Some years and counselling experiences later, a university administrative officer quietly teared up reading the dedication to our son, when I finally submitted the thesis.

Australian universities in the mid-1990s were transitioning to rely less on government funding and more on revenue from tuition fees. Competition between staff and the beginning of what (Smyth et al. 2017) calls neoliberal driven toxic university environments manifested with an accusation of plagiarism levelled at me. This took some time and ombudsman interventions before all accusations were dropped as manifestly unfounded. This experience fuelled an intense distaste for research conducted in toxic, politically motivated university environments. I was no longer concerned that I didn't belong, because I discovered that I did not want to belong in a quite ruthless sector.

However, my doctoral research was quite well received and led to significant grants including an elite post-doctoral research award to work with industry. This research-only position outside of university politics allowed me to validate the artificial intelligence and law modelling methods I pioneered. I had published some dozens of journal papers and won many prestigious grants. I was beginning to bask in the *Ribbon* rewards. However, fearing a return to the politics of a university research environment when the post-doctoral grants ended, I seized on an opportunity to spin out a start-up company based at a regional university's technology park, and dedicated my efforts to advancing the research so that artificial intelligence and machine learning could be directed to enhance justice; an incentive I now recognise as a *Moral* factor. The promise of *Gold* in the early start-up was palpable. Write ups in the *The Economist, MIT Technology Review, invited keynotes*, more Australian Research Council grants and prestigious publications continued to fan the *Ribbons*. The technical challenge of building cutting edge, smart systems while supervising my own doctoral students fuelled the *Puzzle* motivators.

The failure to attract investors led to cash flow issues and forced the closure of the start-up and though the company years were exhilarating, I needed to reflect on my next move. Looking back on the previous decade of research I saw that the thing that gave me the greatest sense of satisfaction was that I had engineered an AI application that made a real difference to under-privileged applicants for legal aid and that my wife and I had two beautiful young children. With a renewed sense of enthusiasm, I stepped up to a full-time academic career at the regional university that was transitioning from a vocational college to a university. I knew this was the worst thing for my *Ribbon* and *Gold* ambitions but the spin-out experience and young children were more compelling. I had a love for teaching and found that I mostly enjoyed seeing students from diverse, often under-privileged backgrounds, grow and succeed. I was part of nascent research centre filled with a diverse and close-knit group of mathematicians and information technology researchers that was remarkably devoid of the backstabbing politics that characterised other university workplaces. Many of the mathematicians had come to the regional university following the collapse of the Soviet Union and themselves were enjoying a setting devoid of the worst of university politics. I felt grateful and intuitively felt it was time to shift my research direction from law to health informatics to cement the fresh start. Working on how emerging technologies could empower patients to participate in their own health and well-being rather than leaving it all up to doctors, was meaningful to me given our first baby's passing. The trend emerging for patients to access medical information on the Internet to make informed choices was originally seen positively (Bauer 2002). Hewlett et al. (2006) had found that patients working collaboratively together with researchers has benefits for all. Over the following decade a review of patient participation in research by Brett et al. (2014) revealed over 60 publications reporting benefits and challenges of having patients work directly with research teams. Although most of the studies reviewed had worked with patients by communicating with a user group rather than directly involving patients in the research team. Nevertheless, evidence was found that this collaboration helped to formulate better research questions, better interpretations of data and better ways to engage with patients. Challenges involved additional time required from all participants, and experiences when trying to make sense of patterns that arose from data analytics exercises.

Since around 2010, fuelled by our experiences with our first child, I have been dismayed by the gulf that exists between communities of diverse medical systems and that health informatics research is almost exclusively directed toward allopathic medicine (Stranieri and Vaughan 2010). Early work to address this with a prominent homeopathy practitioner and researcher colleague was promising but ended abruptly when my university withdraw his unpaid affiliation following concern at the executive level that the association might threaten medical grant applications submitted by clinical schools. Preliminary work with Ayurvedic medicine informatics (Stranieri et al. 2017) and Traditional Chinese Medicine informatics failed to lead to publications in top-ranked journals or the cross-disciplinary collaborations we envisaged. Our son had developed a chronic illness during his teenage years and was forced out of secondary school. His valiant efforts to home school himself while managing his condition demanded all the focus we could muster. The research skills were very useful in keeping up with the latest research but no cure was in sight. I was a mid-career research then motivated in a curious way by *Gold*, *Ribbons*, *Puzzle* and *Moral* factors and, at the same time, by none of them.

Designing technologies to enhance multi-disciplinary group reasoning (Sharma et al. 2016) and visualisation to empower patients in shared care (Sharma et al. 2018) and understanding group clinical reasoning on ward rounds (Perversi et al. 2018) are all research directions driven by a sense that our technologies ought to be directed to empowering patients to interact meaningfully with health care professionals. The university sector in Australia has continued to grow more toxic but this has fuelled an interest in deliberative reasoning and how technologies can enhance ideal forms of dialogue (Yearwood and Stranieri 2012). An entry into research into remote patient monitoring was motivated by the passing of my colleagues father

(Allami et al. 2017; Balasubramanian et al. 2015). This has led to another start-up company addressing the problem that periodic vital sign measurement misses many patient deteriorations compared with continuous, remote monitoring (Prgomet et al. 2016).

The regional university has undergone numerous major re-structures in the last decade and the convivial research centre has closed. Our son successfully taught himself the secondary school curriculum as a correspondence student and is conducting doctoral research on a condition similar to his own. Our daughter is stridently pursuing a career in film production after a most interesting Masters' exegesis.

In summary, I can see that key beliefs and life events including my transfer into an Arts degree, years of blue-collar jobs, my journey into accepting myself as a researcher, the loss of our first child, a thorough distaste for toxicity in university workplaces, the enjoyment in seeing diverse students succeed and an urge to direct our technologies to enhance health and well-being, have led to different decisions at different points in time. The *Gold, Ribbon, Puzzle* and *Moral* motivating factors were present in one way or another; however, the relative importance and intensity was mediated by experiences in my life outside research at each juncture. Many of the research directions I have pursued and major decisions can be seen to flow directly from embodied cognition, the combination of the intuitive and the rational in the specific contexts that they occurred.

3   Concluding Remarks

According to Nowotny (2010), the modern era is characterised by a society-wide fascination and quest for innovation. For millennia, research was largely performed through universities although many great and notable advances were made outside of university settings. Newton's calculus and the laws of gravity were discovered during a 2-year period while he worked at home during the 1665–1666 plague as Cambridge University was closed (Moore 2018). Darwin's voyage on the Beagle and subsequent interests were driven by his innate curiosity (Berra 2008). The emergence in the last century of state and private Research Technology Organisations (RTO) that aim to generate commercial outcomes engaged researchers who were not distracted by teaching (Suominen et al. 2021). Concerns that academics were becoming more interested in commercialisation and motivated by profit raised by Vallas and Kleinman (2008) led to an interest in studying the researchers' motivations.

That researchers are motivated by financial rewards, recognition, curiosity and a desire to make a contribution the so-called *Gold, Ribbons, Puzzle* and *Moral* motivating factors is taken as the foundation for the exercise in introspection here. However, the way in which life events and situations impact these categories is explored with an introspection over a research career spanning 25 years in artificial intelligence and law, and health informatics.

References

Abma TA. Dialogue and deliberation: new approaches to including patients in setting health and healthcare research agendas. Action Res. 2019;17(4):429–50.

Allami R, Stranieri A, Balasubramanian V, Jelinek HF. A count data model for heart rate variability forecasting and premature ventricular contraction detection. SIViP. 2017;2017:1–9.

Atta-Owusu K, Fitjar RD. What motivates academics for external engagement? Exploring the effects of motivational drivers and organizational fairness. Sci Public Policy. 2022;49(2):201–18.

Balasubramanian V, Stranieri A, Kaur R. Appa: assistive patient monitoring cloud platform for active healthcare applications. Paper presented at the Proceedings of the 9th International Conference on Ubiquitous Information Management and Communication. 2015.

Baptista A, Frick L, Holley K, Remmik M, Tesch J, Âkerlind G. The doctorate as an original contribution to knowledge: considering relationships between originality, creativity, and innovation. Frontline Learn Res. 2015;3(3):55–67.

Bauer KA. Using the Internet to empower patients and to develop partnerships with clinicians. World Hosp Health Serv. 2002;38(2):2–10.

Bellini-Leite SC. Dual process theory: embodied and predictive; symbolic and classical. Front Psychol. 2022;13:805386.

Berra TM. Charles Darwin: the concise story of an extraordinary man. Baltimore: Johns Hopkins University Press; 2008.

Brett J, Staniszewska S, Mockford C, Herron-Marx S, Hughes J, Tysall C, Suleman R. Mapping the impact of patient and public involvement on health and social care research: a systematic review. Health Expect. 2014;17(5):637–50. https://doi.org/10.1111/j.1369-7625.2012.00795.x.

Buckholtz JW, Asplund CL, Dux PE, Zald DH, Gore JC, Jones OD, Marois R. The neural correlates of third-party punishment. Neuron. 2008;60(5):930–40.

Burkart T. Dialogic introspection—a method of investigating experience. Hum Arenas. 2018;1(2):167–90.

Clarke CL, Wilkinson H, Watson J, Wilcockson J, Kinnaird L, Williamson T. A seat around the table: participatory data analysis with people living with dementia. Qual Health Res. 2018;28(9):1421–33.

Evans JSB, Stanovich KE. Dual-process theories of higher cognition: advancing the debate. Perspect Psychol Sci. 2013;8(3):223–41.

Hewlett S, Wit MD, Richards P, Quest E, Hughes R, Heiberg T, Kirwan J. Patients and professionals as research partners: challenges, practicalities, and benefits. Arthritis Care Res. 2006;55(4):676–80.

Joynson C, Leyser O. The culture of scientific research. F1000Research. 2015;4:66.

Kahneman D. Thinking fast and slow. New York: Straus and Giroux; 2011.

Kirwan JR, De Wit M, Frank L, Haywood KL, Salek S, Brace-McDonnell S, Guillemin F. Emerging guidelines for patient engagement in research. Value Health. 2017;20(3):481–6.

Kwasnicka D, Dombrowski SU, White M, Sniehotta F. Theoretical explanations for maintenance of behaviour change: a systematic review of behaviour theories. Health Psychol Rev. 2016;10(3):277–96.

Lam A. Academic scientists and knowledge commercialization: self-determination and diverse motivations. In: Incentives and performance. Cham: Springer; 2015. p. 173–87.

Moore JC. A brief history of universities. Cham: Springer; 2018.

Nowotny H. Insatiable curiosity: innovation in a fragile future. Cambridge: MIT Press; 2010.

Parkman A. The imposter phenomenon in higher education: Incidence and impact. J Higher Educ Theory Pract. 2016;16(1):51–60.

Perversi P, Yearwood J, Bellucci E, Stranieri A, Warren J, Burstein F, Wolff A. Exploring reasoning mechanisms in ward rounds: a critical realist multiple case study. BMC Health Serv Res. 2018;18(1):643. https://doi.org/10.1186/s12913-018-3446-6.

Pinder C, Vermeulen J, Cowan BR, Beale R. Digital behaviour change interventions to break and form habits. ACM Trans Comp Hum Interact. 2018;25(3):1–66.

Prgomet M, Cardona-Morrell M, Nicholson M, Lake R, Long J, Westbrook J, Hillman K. Vital signs monitoring on general wards: clinical staff perceptions of current practices and the planned introduction of continuous monitoring technology. Int J Qual Health Care. 2016;28(4):515–21.

Riggare S. Patient researchers—the missing link? Nat Med. 2020;26(10):1507. https://doi.org/10.1038/s41591-020-1080-4.

Sharma V, Stranieri A, Burstein F, Warren J, Daly S, Patterson L, Wolff A. Group decision making in health care: a case study of multidisciplinary meetings. J Decis Syst. 2016;25(1):476–85.

Sharma V, Stranieri A, Firmin S, Mays H, Burstein F. Approaches for the visualization of health information. Paper presented at the Proceedings of the Australasian Computer Science Week Multiconference. 2018:1–9.

Smyth J, Toxic University: Zombie Leadership, Academic Rock Stars and Neoliberal Ideology Cham: Springer; 2017.

Strack F, Deutsch R. Reflective and impulsive determinants of social behavior. Personal Soc Psychol Rev. 2004;8(3):220–47.

Stranieri A, Vaughan S. Coalescing medical systems: a challenge for health informatics in a global world. Stud Health Technol Inform. 2010;161:159–68.

Stranieri A, Butler-Henderson K, Sahama T, Perera PK, Da Silva JL, Pelonio D, Raghavachar D. A visual grid to digitally record an Ayurvedic Prakriti assessment; a first step toward integrated electronic health records. J Tradit Complement Med. 2017;7(2):264.

Suominen A, Kauppinen H, Hyytinen K. 'Gold', 'Ribbon' or 'Puzzle': what motivates researchers to work in research and technology organizations. Technol Forecast Soc Chang. 2021;170:120882.

Vallas SP, Kleinman DL. Contradiction, convergence and the knowledge economy: the confluence of academic and commercial biotechnology. Soc Econ Rev. 2008;6(2):283–311.

Van De Burgwal LH, Hendrikse R, Claassen E. Aiming for impact: differential effect of motivational drivers on effort and performance in knowledge valorisation. Sci Public Policy. 2019;46(5):747–62.

Yearwood J, Stranieri A. Approaches for community decision making and collective reasoning: knowledge technology support. Hershey: IGI Global; 2012.